Coping with Anaemia

Dr Tom Smith has been writing since 1977, after spending six years in general practice and seven years in medical research. He wrote the 'Doctor, Doctor' column in *The Guardian* on Saturdays, and has written three humorous books, *Doctor, Have You Got a Minute?*, *A Seaside Practice* and *Going Loco*, all published by Short Books. His other books for Sheldon Press include *Heart Attacks: Prevent and Survive*, *Living with Alzheimer's Disease*, *Overcoming Back Pain*, *Coping with Bowel Cancer*, *Coping with Heartburn and Reflux*, *Coping with Age-related Memory Loss*, *101 Questions to Ask Your Doctor*, *How to Get the Best from Your Doctor*, *Coping with Kidney Disease*, *Osteoporosis: Prevent and Treat*, *Coping Successfully with Prostate Cancer* and *Reducing Your Risk of Dementia*.

Overcoming Common Problems Series

Selected titles

A full list of titles is available from Sheldon Press,
36 Causton Street, London SW1P 4ST and on our website at
www.sheldonpress.co.uk

101 Questions to Ask Your Doctor
Dr Tom Smith

Asperger Syndrome in Adults
Dr Ruth Searle

The Assertiveness Handbook
Mary Hartley

Assertiveness: Step by step
Dr Windy Dryden and Daniel Constantinou

Backache: What you need to know
Dr David Delvin

Birth Over 35
Sheila Kitzinger

Body Language: What you need to know
David Cohen

Bulimia, Binge-eating and their Treatment
Professor J. Hubert Lacey, Dr Bryony Bamford
and Amy Brown

The Cancer Survivor's Handbook
Dr Terry Priestman

The Chronic Pain Diet Book
Neville Shone

Cider Vinegar
Margaret Hills

Coeliac Disease: What you need to know
Alex Gazzola

Coping Successfully with Pain
Neville Shone

Coping Successfully with Prostate Cancer
Dr Tom Smith

Coping Successfully with Shyness
Margaret Oakes, Professor Robert Bor
Dr Carina Eriksen

Coping Successfully with Ulcerative Colitis
Peter Cartwright

Coping Successfully with Varicose Veins
Christine Craggs-Hinton

Coping Successfully with Your Hiatus Hernia
Dr Tom Smith

Coping Successfully with Your Irritable Bowel
Rosemary Nicol

Coping When Your Child Has Cerebral Palsy
Jill Eckersley

Coping with Anaemia
Dr Tom Smith

Coping with Asthma in Adults
Mark Greener

Coping with Birth Trauma and Postnatal Depression
Lucy Jolin

Coping with Bowel Cancer
Dr Tom Smith

Coping with Bronchitis and Emphysema
Dr Tom Smith

Coping with Candida
Shirley Trickett

Coping with Chemotherapy
Dr Terry Priestman

Coping with Chronic Fatigue
Trudie Chalder

Coping with Coeliac Disease
Karen Brody

Coping with Diverticulitis
Peter Cartwright

Coping with Drug Problems in the Family
Lucy Jolin

Coping with Dyspraxia
Jill Eckersley

Coping with Early-onset Dementia
Jill Eckersley

Coping with Eating Disorders and Body Image
Christine Craggs-Hinton

Coping with Envy
Dr Windy Dryden

Coping with Gout
Christine Craggs-Hinton

Coping with Headaches and Migraine
Alison Frith

Coping with Heartburn and Reflux
Dr Tom Smith

Coping with Life after Stroke
Dr Mareeni Raymond

Coping with Life's Challenges: Moving on from adversity
Dr Windy Dryden

Overcoming Common Problems Series

Coping with Manipulation: When others blame you for their feelings
Dr Windy Dryden

Coping with Obsessive Compulsive Disorder
Professor Kevin Gournay, Rachel Piper
and Professor Paul Rogers

Coping with Phobias and Panic
Professor Kevin Gournay

Coping with PMS
Dr Farah Ahmed and Dr Emma Cordle

Coping with Polycystic Ovary Syndrome
Christine Craggs-Hinton

Coping with the Psychological Effects of Cancer
Professor Robert Bor, Dr Carina Eriksen
and Ceilidh Stapelkamp

Coping with Radiotherapy
Dr Terry Priestman

Coping with Rheumatism and Arthritis
Dr Keith Souter

Coping with Snoring and Sleep Apnoea
Jill Eckersley

Coping with Stomach Ulcers
Dr Tom Smith

Coping with Suicide
Maggie Helen

Coping with Type 2 Diabetes
Susan Elliot-Wright

Depressive Illness: The curse of the strong
Dr Tim Cantopher

Divorce and Separation: A legal guide for all couples
Dr Mary Welstead

Dying for a Drink
Dr Tim Cantopher

Dynamic Breathing: How to manage your asthma
Dinah Bradley and Tania Clifton-Smith

Epilepsy: Complementary and alternative treatments
Dr Sallie Baxendale

The Fertility Handbook
Dr Philippa Kaye

The Fibromyalgia Healing Diet
Christine Craggs-Hinton

Free Yourself from Depression
Colin and Margaret Sutherland

A Guide to Anger Management
Mary Hartley

The Heart Attack Survival Guide
Mark Greener

Helping Children Cope with Anxiety
Jill Eckersley

Helping Children Cope with Grief
Rosemary Wells

High-risk Body Size: Take control of your weight
Dr Funké Baffour

How to Beat Worry and Stress
Dr David Delvin

How to Cope with Difficult People
Alan Houel and Christian Godefroy

How to Develop Inner Strength
Dr Windy Dryden

How to Live with a Control Freak
Barbara Baker

How to Lower Your Blood Pressure: And keep it down
Christine Craggs-Hinton

How to Manage Chronic Fatigue
Christine Craggs-Hinton

Hysterectomy: Is it right for you?
Janet Wright

The IBS Healing Plan
Theresa Cheung

Let's Stay Together: A guide to lasting relationships
Jane Butterworth

Living with Angina
Dr Tom Smith

Living with Asperger Syndrome
Dr Joan Gomez

Living with Autism
Fiona Marshall

Living with Bipolar Disorder
Dr Neel Burton

Living with Crohn's Disease
Dr Joan Gomez

Living with Eczema
Jill Eckersley

Living with Fibromyalgia
Christine Craggs-Hinton

Living with Gluten Intolerance
Jane Feinmann

Living with IBS
Nuno Ferreira and David T. Gillanders

Living with Loss and Grief
Julia Tugendhat

Living with Osteoarthritis
Dr Patricia Gilbert

Living with Osteoporosis
Dr Joan Gomez

Living with Physical Disability and Amputation
Dr Keren Fisher

Overcoming Common Problems Series

**Living with a Problem Drinker:
Your survival guide**
Rolande Anderson

Living with Rheumatoid Arthritis
Philippa Pigache

Living with Schizophrenia
Dr Neel Burton and Dr Phil Davison

Living with a Seriously Ill Child
Dr Jan Aldridge

Living with a Stoma
Professor Craig A. White

Living with Tinnitus and Hyperacusis
Dr Laurence McKenna, Dr David Baguley
and Dr Don McFerran

Losing a Child
Linda Hurcombe

Losing a Parent
Fiona Marshall

**Making Sense of Trauma: How to tell
your story**
Dr Nigel C. Hunt and Dr Sue McHale

Menopause in Perspective
Philippa Pigache

Motor Neurone Disease: A family affair
Dr David Oliver

The Multiple Sclerosis Diet Book
Tessa Buckley

Natural Treatments for Arthritis
Christine Craggs-Hinton

Osteoporosis: Prevent and treat
Dr Tom Smith

Overcome Your Fear of Flying
Professor Robert Bor, Dr Carina Eriksen
and Margaret Oakes

Overcoming Agoraphobia
Melissa Murphy

Overcoming Anorexia
Professor J. Hubert Lacey, Christine
Craggs-Hinton and Kate Robinson

Overcoming Emotional Abuse
Susan Elliot-Wright

**Overcoming Gambling: A guide for problem
and compulsive gamblers**
Philip Mawer

Overcoming Hurt
Dr Windy Dryden

Overcoming Jealousy
Dr Windy Dryden

Overcoming Loneliness
Alice Muir

**Overcoming Panic and Related Anxiety
Disorders**
Margaret Hawkins

Overcoming Procrastination
Dr Windy Dryden

Overcoming Shyness and Social Anxiety
Dr Ruth Searle

Overcoming Tiredness and Exhaustion
Fiona Marshall

**The Pain Management Handbook:
Your personal guide**
Neville Shone

Reducing Your Risk of Dementia
Dr Tom Smith

**Self-discipline: How to get it
and how to keep it**
Dr Windy Dryden

The Self-Esteem Journal
Alison Waines

Sinusitis: Steps to healing
Dr Paul Carson

Stammering: Advice for all ages
Renée Byrne and Louise Wright

Stress-related Illness
Dr Tim Cantopher

Ten Steps to Positive Living
Dr Windy Dryden

**Therapy for Beginners: How to get the best out
of counselling**
Professor Robert Bor, Sheila Gill and Anne Stokes

Think Your Way to Happiness
Dr Windy Dryden and Jack Gordon

**Tranquillizers and Antidepressants: When to
take them, how to stop**
Professor Malcolm Lader

**Transforming Eight Deadly Emotions
into Healthy Ones**
Dr Windy Dryden

The Traveller's Good Health Guide
Dr Ted Lankester

Treating Arthritis Diet Book
Margaret Hills

Treating Arthritis: The drug-free way
Margaret Hills and Christine Horner

Treating Arthritis: More ways to a drug-free life
Margaret Hills

Treating Arthritis: The supplements guide
Julia Davies

Understanding Obsessions and Compulsions
Dr Frank Tallis

Understanding Traumatic Stress
Dr Nigel Hunt and Dr Sue McHale

The User's Guide to the Male Body
Jim Pollard

When Someone You Love Has Dementia
Susan Elliot-Wright

Overcoming Common Problems

Coping with Anaemia

DR TOM SMITH

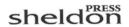

sheldon PRESS

First published in Great Britain in 2012

Sheldon Press
36 Causton Street
London SW1P 4ST
www.sheldonpress.co.uk

British Library Cataloguing-in-Publication Data
A catalogue record for this book is available from the British Library

ISBN 978–1–84709–232–8
eBook ISBN 978–1–84709–233–5

Typeset by Caroline Waldron, Wirral, Cheshire
First printed in Great Britain by Ashford Colour Press
Subsequently digitally printed in Great Britain

Contents

Introduction   ix

Note to the reader   xviii

1   Our healthy blood   1

2   Some people with blood-loss anaemia   5

3   Why we need iron   21

4   Anaemia in pregnancy   43

5   Folic acid-deficiency anaemia and pernicious anaemia   53

6   Anaemia in older people   64

7   Anaemia in arthritis and cancer   74

8   Sickle-cell anaemia and thalassaemia   80

9   Some less common anaemias   92

10   Some golden bullets   99

References   102

Index   105

Introduction

It's odd that there haven't been previous books for the general public on anaemia, because it is the commonest physical abnormality of human beings worldwide. Note that I didn't describe anaemia as an 'illness' or a 'disease', because it is neither. Rather, it is an indication of some underlying problem that has led to it. Medically speaking, it is a sign of an illness, not a diagnosis in itself. The many illnesses that cause anaemia, and how we recognize them and treat them, are what this book is about.

So when a doctor finds that you are anaemic, he or she needs to find the cause and correct it. Simply trying to treat anaemia without finding that cause – for example, just pre-scribing iron tablets – is poor medicine and may even be dangerous for you. At the very least, though it might help for a while, it delays and can unnecessarily complicate your eventual diagnosis. At worst, it may even be lethal. So if you think you are anaemic, you need good medical support and expertise. It isn't a condition that you should try to treat yourself.

Nor should you assume that you are anaemic because you look pale, are always tired, and get easily exhausted and breathless when you exercise. None of these symptoms are exclusive to anaemia: in fact, some people can be very severely anaemic and still feel reasonably well. When they find out they are anaemic, they are often astonished.

So let's start with a definition. 'Anaemia' means 'lack of blood'. If we take the ancient Greek literally it means 'absence of blood', but that's not helpful. A person whose blood has been completely drained is dead, not anaemic. So how much lower than average has your blood level got to fall before you are labelled as anaemic?

You would think I would have an easy answer, but I don't. Two centuries ago, when doctors, tragically, used blood-letting as a main part of their systems of treatment, they would note that in some people the blood was 'thin, pale and watery'. The word 'anaemia' was born then. Naturally, with each new bleeding session, the blood became thinner and even more watery. It was odd that the doctors of the time didn't relate their regular bleeding sessions to the worsening of their patients' illnesses, and even to their deaths. Read the accounts of the final few days of King Charles II to marvel at the relative ignorance of the doctors of the time.

Happily, we have progressed a lot since then. We have very accurate, automated blood-analysing machines that measure exactly how densely packed your blood is with red cells (technically erythrocytes), how much haemoglobin (the pigment that makes the blood red) is in each cell, and how concentrated it is. They also measure the size and shape of the cells, and what percentage of them are fresh 'young' red cells. (They are called reticulocytes, about which there is more later.) Your sample will be centrifuged down to show what proportions of your blood are composed of red cells, of white cells (leukocytes) and of the plasma, the clear fluid in which they float. All this will make sense as you read on. The point of mentioning them now is to introduce you to the idea that anaemia isn't just a deficiency of iron: it's a much more complex condition that needs more than the simple measurement of haemoglobin (the finger-tip needle-prick test your doctor uses as a first check) to understand and define it, and then to treat it.

Even when we know your haemoglobin level, that doesn't mean that below a certain well-defined line you are definitely anaemic. It's accepted, for example, that women on average have lower haemoglobin levels than men: a whole chapter of this book, on anaemia in pregnancy, is devoted to this difference. If you are pregnant, the excess fluid you have in your body, diluting your blood, makes a haemoglobin level that is even lower than usual completely acceptable. For many years pregnant women were given iron tablets unnecessarily because their lower haemoglobin levels were misinterpreted as anaemia. We know better now.

Much depends, too, on where you live. People who live in the high hills and mountains have higher haemoglobin levels than people at sea level. That's a normal adaptation to the need to gather more oxygen from the lighter atmosphere. When their very high haemoglobin levels drop they are in trouble: a Himalayan Sherpa with a haemoglobin that has dropped into the normal range for sea-level dwellers is considered anaemic and a concern to his doctor.

Then there are people whose haemoglobin levels are naturally at the high or low edges of the normal for their community. Their doctors would start to worry if, say, someone recorded previously as having a high haemoglobin, say of 15 grams per decilitre, now has one of 13. Although 13 is still 'normal' for the rest of the population, such a drop suggests blood loss and a relative anaemia compared to that person's previous levels. We need to identify the site of the loss and its cause.

So anaemia is not a precise diagnosis in which there are strict cut-off points that apply to every person. Along with our assessment of your blood results, we need to take into account your past history and tests and make a judgement on whether or not the results are normal or abnormal. There is no finely defined border between the two – unless a result is so far out of line that it is obviously the result of serious disease. Having a much lower than normal haemoglobin has to be looked upon as just as much a sign of illness as, say, pain, loss of weight, a disturbance in your heart rhythm, indigestion or a high blood sugar. But it says nothing about the underlying cause.

Why do we need our blood in the first place? That red cell pigment, haemoglobin, picks up oxygen from the air in our lungs, combines with it, and carries it throughout our circulation to the tissues, where the combination loosens and the oxygen is given up, to be transported to wherever it is needed in plentiful supply. In the tissues – the skin, the brain, every organ and every system – the oxygen is exchanged for carbon dioxide, and the red cells and plasma carry that back to the lungs, where the cycle begins again.

Our tissues use up the oxygen as our 'fuel': it burns up glucose to make the energy we need to keep alive. Without an adequate mass of haemoglobin (which is normally only present inside our red cells) we cannot deliver enough oxygen for our needs. The problem is that we don't notice a small slow fall in our haemoglobin levels: our bodies adjust to the change by subtle increases in our heart rate, so that the blood is pumped faster from lungs to tissues. The heart beats a little bit faster, so that the red cells visit the lungs a little more often, to pick up and deliver the extra oxygen that we need.

That process is sometimes so hidden from our consciousness that, if it occurs slowly over a long time, we don't begin to notice it until we may have lost two-thirds or even more of our haemoglobin. In one type of anaemia in which this happens, pernicious anaemia (about which more later), the haemoglobin level may even drop from its normal of 13 to 15 grams per decilitre of blood to around 5 grams per decilitre before sufferers notice that they are breathing faster and are much weaker than they used to be. Oddly, they don't necessarily feel tired: often the lack of oxygen can make them over-alert and they can't get to sleep.

So although it's a common belief that we should know when we are anaemic, we usually don't. Family doctors like me, looking back on our patients over the years, will remember far more of them who were discovered to be anaemic by chance, usually on a routine blood test, than because they were showing obvious symptoms. What alerts us to taking the blood tests in such cases is described in Chapter 2, in a series of patients I have known over the years. You may recognize yourself among them.

The converse of this is that many people think that they are anaemic when they are not. It's a widely held belief that tiredness, listlessness, breathlessness on simple exercise and pale skin, eyes and fingernails are sure signs of anaemia. Although they may be, they are often signs of other problems instead. Breathlessness, for example, may be a sign of heart or lung failure, in which case you may even have an excess of red cells in your blood. We make the extra cells to provide more oxygen when our hearts can't pump the blood around as efficiently as they should. Or our lungs, thickened and stiffened perhaps by chronic lung disease, can't easily transfer the amount of oxygen we need across to our red cells, so we make more of them in order to pick up as much as possible.

Looking pale isn't a reliable indicator of anaemia either. You may look pale because the blood vessels just under the surface of the skin have narrowed: you can be cold and pale, but completely healthy and not anaemic. Smokers look pale and pasty because of this lack of blood flow through the skin (the nicotine narrows their small arteries), but they aren't necessarily anaemic. When doctors pull down your lower eyelids to look at the colour of the skin behind them, they may note that they are paler than usual but that, too, can deceive. Pale eyes may not reflect your red-cell level, and red eyes can even hide anaemia. And if you have a darker skin tone, it is difficult to know if you have become paler than you were. So we don't depend any more on looks if we wish to make an accurate diagnosis. That blood test is the only true criterion.

The only effective way to tell the difference between those who are anaemic and those who aren't is to examine their blood. There is no substitute for measurement, and no reason ever to treat anyone for anaemia without knowing what we are dealing with. As you read on, you will quickly understand the importance of this fundamental aspect of medicine.

Once you have been given the diagnosis of anaemia, it is only the start of our investigations. We need to find out why this has happened to you. To do that we first must ask you questions that may give a clue to why your blood count is low.

The cause of anaemia should, in theory, be relatively easy to discover. Blood counts fall for one of five general reasons:

- We are not eating enough of the correct foods to make the fresh red blood cells that we need.
- We are eating enough, but are not, for some reason, digesting the materials we need to make the red cells.
- We are eating and digesting the correct foods, but for some reason our bone marrow is not converting them into red blood cells.
- We are eating and digesting normally and our bone marrow is normal, but we are losing more blood each day than the body can replace in new red cells.
- We are making enough red cells, but they aren't lasting as long as the three months or so that normal red cells last.

In more developed societies the first cause is rare: our problem is more likely to be eating too much than to be limiting our food intake so severely that we can't form enough red cells. However, for a small minority of people on faddy or very restricted diets, anaemia is a risk they seem to be prepared to take. Starvation in countries where the agriculture and/

or the economy has failed is a different matter: it leads to far more than simple anaemia. It also leads to lack of protein, carbohydrate and fat. Simply topping up with iron would not scratch the surface of the problem.

Poor digestion from bowel and stomach disorders does cause anaemia, but most people with them show other symptoms, like abdominal pain and bloating, that indicate that there is a wider problem as well as their anaemia. One exception to this is pernicious anaemia, in which the stomach wall can't form the chemical (called intrinsic factor) that is essential to digesting vitamin B12. Without it anaemia becomes inevitable: one chapter is set aside for this form of anaemia and a similar illness caused by deficiency of another of the B vitamins, folic acid.

Bone marrow failure is a much rarer cause of anaemia, but has become important in the last few years because it can be a disastrous side effect of some modern drugs, so it, too, deserves a mention. The anaemias that come with chronic kidney disease (much commoner than we thought a few years ago) and some cancers are also the result of poor bone marrow function. Happily, we have learned how to reverse them, and one chapter will be devoted to them.

Anaemias caused by loss of blood are by far the commonest form. Only a few millilitres of blood need to be lost every day for anaemia to develop. Our bone marrow can't increase its production by enough to restore all of the lost red cells, and gradually we become anaemic. As explained above, the loss may be so slight that we don't feel any discomfort or show any signs of anaemia. Yet it is vital to identify it. Most cases of bowel cancer are initially identified from discovering that an otherwise healthy adult either is anaemic or is passing microscopic amounts of blood in his or her stool. I have a strong personal reason for writing this: in 2008 this was exactly how my own bowel cancer was diagnosed. Happily it was caught in plenty of time, I had the appropriate surgery, and, writing in 2012, I'm still clear of the disease.

The blood loss may be from higher in the gut, say from a stomach ulcer, or from active inflammatory bowel disease, such as Crohn's disease or ulcerative colitis. You may even be made anaemic from something as simple as a haemorrhoid (pile). I cover all these causes later in the book. Or it can be the result of heavy periods. Many women take heavy periods for granted: they may well, unknowingly, be anaemic because of them. Blood may also be leaking from your bladder: it's easy to miss it, as it doesn't necessarily show up as red urine. So when you are asked to attend your local surgery or health clinic for your regular well-man or well-woman visit, please do so. Finding that you have anaemia at such times may well be the first and even only sign of an underlying illness that could be a threat. The blood, urine and stool tests taken at these times may save your life.

The last category, in which your red cells don't survive long enough in the bloodstream to keep up your haemoglobin levels, is much less common. Sometimes the fault lies in the red cells self-destructing because of an inherited flaw in their make-up. The most famous case is, of course, that of George III (portrayed brilliantly in the film *The Madness of King George*). In other cases the cells break up in a process called haemolysis: I cover that too, later.

Chapter 1 explains what we look for in a normal blood sample. It goes on to describe how your doctor suspects and diagnoses anaemia. It lists the tests and the results in the common anaemias. Please don't skip it: it is important that you understand them, so that you and your doctor can work together to restore your blood to normality.

From Chapter 2 onwards I describe a series of patients, taken from my own experience, with anaemias of different causes, and how they were managed. I start with the more common conditions, and each succeeding chapter describes a particular type of anaemia, how it is diagnosed and how it is treated. They include some of the rarer anaemias, such as sickle-cell anaemia. This is a consequence of inherited changes in the red blood cells that developed many generations ago as a form of resistance to malaria, but rather than a blessing they are now a problem to their 'owners', who are no longer exposed to malaria-carrying mosquitoes. As our society becomes more cosmopolitan and international, we are meeting people from tropical and subtropical countries who carry the trait and need expert help.

I finish the book with some 'golden bullets' on anaemias, their facts and fallacies. There is huge pressure today to persuade people, even when they are normally healthy, to take extra vitamins, minerals and other food supplements in order to avoid anaemias and other possible forms of ill health. Recent studies strongly suggest that they are more likely to be harmful than beneficial: I have included what is now the mainstream medical thinking on them as part of the final chapter.

Note to the reader

This book is not intended to replace advice from your doctor. Consult your pharmacist or doctor if you believe you have any of the symptoms described, and if you think you might need medical help.

1

Our healthy blood

Before we can understand anaemia we need to know about the blood in normal health. As partly explained in the introduction, our basic unit of blood – what makes it red – is the red cell, or **erythrocyte**. Erythrocytes make up around 45 per cent of our blood: when it is spun in a centrifuge the red cells separate out in the lower half of the tube, showing the proportion of the sample that is composed of red cells, and the plasma above it. This proportion is called the **haematocrit**, about which more later. Lying on top of the red cells, in a very thin layer below the base of the almost transparent plasma, is a very thin whitish disc. In this disc are the white blood cells, or **leukocytes**. The red cells outnumber them, normally by around 1,000 times.

There are around 5 million red cells and around 5,000 white cells per microlitre (a microlitre is a thousandth of a millilitre, so is a tiny drop on a microscope slide) of blood in a healthy person. But simply counting the number of red cells isn't enough. The crucial element inside the red cells – the substance that combines with oxygen in the lungs and carries it to the tissues and organs, where it is released for them to use in producing energy – is the pigment **haemoglobin**. You may have a normal number of red cells, but there may not be enough haemoglobin inside them – or the haemoglobin itself may be abnormal and not able to deal with the oxygen as efficiently as it should. In either case you can be just as anaemic as if you had lost a high proportion of your red cells.

In some anaemias, such as pernicious anaemia and alcohol-overuse anaemia, your red cells may be much larger than normal but contain far less haemoglobin than you need. So despite having bigger than normal red cells, you may still be in an anaemic state.

The shape of the red cell is crucial too. The normal red cell is a disc with a thickened outer edge and a thinner centre. I liken them to the fruit gums we used to have when we were children, the ones that were sold in tubes. That shape is important because it has the optimum surface structure for picking up and releasing oxygen, but is still flexible and deformable enough for the cells to squeeze through the narrowest of blood vessels, allowing the blood to flow freely from the arteries through the capillaries (the smallest blood vessels in which the oxygen exchange takes place), into the veins and back to the heart and lungs. In some forms of anaemia, such as sickle-cell anaemia, oddly shaped red cells make this process much more difficult, and the blood is 'stickier' and more likely to block the flow in the smallest blood vessels.

By now you will realize that a simple blood count must take in much more than the number of red cells in your blood. If you have been told you are anaemic, your blood report will list a host of figures that will not only go a long way to explaining what is wrong but will point to its probable causes. If you would like to know more, next time you visit your doctor ask if you can discuss the details of your report. That is only useful, of course, if you understand what the various figures mean. Table 1 shows the standard measurements and their normal values, so that you can compare your own with them and understand why your doctor has made your particular diagnosis. In later chapters on specific types of anaemia, I will repeatedly refer back to this table.

Table 1 Normal blood test results

	Women	Men
Red cell count in adults	4 to 5.5 million per microlitre	4.5 to 6.5 million per microlitre
Haemoglobin concentration	11.5 to 16.5 grams per 100 millilitres (decilitre)	13.5 to 18.0 grams per decilitre
Haematocrit	35 to 47 per cent	40 to 54 per cent
Red cell volume (mean corpuscular volume or MCV)	76 to 95 cubic micrometres (a micrometre is a thousandth of a millimetre)	
Red cell diameter	6.7 to 7.7 micrometres	
Reticulocyte* count	0.2 to 2 per cent of the total red cell numbers	

*Reticulocytes are newly formed red cells that have just been released into the bloodstream. Mature red cells have a clear, smooth, red appearance, with no blemishes inside them. Reticulocytes have small filament-like structures inside them, easily picked out by eye or by auto-analyser machines. How many can be counted in a blood film is important: if they make up more than 2 per cent of the total number of red cells, it means that the marrow has increased its red cell production, almost certainly to replace excess loss of blood. A higher than normal reticulocyte count strongly suggests continuing blood loss and an overactive marrow that is trying to replace it, and the site of this loss must be identified.

It takes the marrow some time to replace lost red cells. Once it has released reticulocytes into the bloodstream, they quickly mature into normal red cells. These last around three months, so that the turnover is only a few per cent per day. In anaemia the marrow steps up its output, but it cannot replace the loss of more than a few millilitres of red cells a day. The reticulocyte count measures the marrow's efforts at doing so. In severe anaemia, reticulocytes can form 10 per cent or more of the total red cells; the higher the count, the more the daily loss.

Don't be put off by the list of results. They look technical, but they are relatively simple to put into context. For example, a count of under 4 million red cells in a woman or under 4.5 million red cells in a man would alert the doctor to the need to investigate further, because something has lowered the patient's red cell numbers into the anaemic range. If that is linked to, say, a haematocrit of below 35 or 40, depending on the patient's gender, but a normal red cell volume and diameter, it is good evidence of probable blood loss. However, if the red cell volume is raised, say to 105 cubic micrometres or above, and the red cell diameter has increased to above 8 micrometres, then we must look for another cause of the anaemia, such as vitamin B12 deficiency or alcoholism.

If the low red cell count is linked to a normal or low reticulocyte count, then the bone marrow is not responding in the usual way to try to replace the loss. That suggests that blood loss is either not the cause or is not the only factor in producing the anaemia. A high reticulocyte count, on the other hand, points to a robust response from the bone marrow, and your doctor will look for chronic bleeding as the cause.

In the next chapter, I use case histories from my own experience as a general practitioner as examples of how blood test results can help to pinpoint the underlying causes of different forms of anaemia. You may find one of these cases resembles your own. Some are very common, but I make no excuse for including causes of anaemia that are rare. In our cosmopolitan society, family doctors are meeting more and more people with illnesses that used to be unique to tropical and subtropical countries. Among them are inherited red blood-cell disorders that lead to anaemia: numbers of British people with them, sometimes among third- and fourth-generation descendants of the original immigrant, are rising. Some may not even know of their family's origin and will be surprised at their diagnosis. You may be among them.

However, the commonest causes of anaemia need the most space, so I start with them.

2

Some people with blood-loss anaemia

The woman who 'just felt off'

Ann Morgan was a farmer's wife. Married for 40 years, with two grown-up children and a busy husband running a hill farm with sheep and beef cattle, she had worked hard physically all her life. Now aged 60, she was expecting to slow down a little, but the economics of running a small farm without help (her husband Bill had had to let his only employee go) did not allow her to do so. Despite Bill cutting down on his stock, she still needed to share his burden. They had not had a holiday for years.

So when she started to feel more tired than before and needed to rest during the day – something unknown in previous years – Ann simply assumed that her age was catching up with her. It was normal, she persuaded herself, to feel less energetic as she grew older. In any case, she couldn't do anything about it: she was too busy to visit me. She would just have to make do and take extra rests when she could grab them. She kept her feelings to herself. She didn't want to trouble Bill about it, as she felt he had enough worries without her adding to them.

It was Ann's sister Jean who alerted me to Ann's illness. Jean lived over 200 miles away, so visited her only once or twice a year. She phoned me after one of these visits, saying that Ann didn't look as ruddy-faced as usual and that she might have lost some weight. More than that, she wasn't her normal jovial and bubbly self, and she had admitted to her sister that she 'just felt off' these days.

I looked up Ann's notes, and was struck by the fact that she hadn't seen a doctor on her own behalf for more than ten years. I knew her only because she was Bill's wife and she had come into the village with him on his regular visits for blood pressure checks. She had not responded to several letters from the practice team asking her to call for a well-woman check. That suggested one of two reasons: she was either in such robust health that she never needed me, or she was wary or frightened of doctor visits and what they might uncover in terms of hidden illness.

I told Ann that I would look in on the farm, on the pretext that I needed to check Bill's blood pressure in his home environment. That wasn't a falsehood: from time to time it's a good idea to do this, as the surgery measurement is often higher than one taken at home. I planned then to raise with Ann how she felt.

Two days later I was with Bill and Ann in their sitting room, with a cup of tea and a scone. Bill's blood pressure had been satisfactory, and Ann protested, when I asked about her, that she was 'fine'.

She didn't look fine. She was pale, and thinner than I remembered her. Despite her protests she seemed anxious, unable to sit still and relax, even in her own home with the cat on her lap. I asked if I could examine her, and she reluctantly agreed.

Although she had been seated for at least ten minutes, her pulse rate was faster than it should have been, at around 90 beats per minute. Her blood pressure was normal, and there was nothing else of any importance to see. Yes, she was pale, but not obviously paler than her husband, who I knew had a haemoglobin of 14 grams per decilitre.

I took a finger-prick sample of blood from Ann and dabbed

it on to a haemoglobin-measuring stick. It read 9 grams per decilitre, far below the normal for any adult, man or woman.

At 60, of course, she was well past her menopause, but I still had to ask about bleeding. There had been none. She sometimes had an ache in the right side of her tummy, she told me, but she was sure that was just wind. That troubled me. Wind, which medically is an accumulation of gas in the bowel, is usually felt in the left side of the abdomen: it is less common on the right, unless something is trapping it there. Pain in the right side plus anaemia and feeling generally unwell added up to the need to investigate urgently.

I felt her abdomen, starting gently on the right side, moving my flat hand across just under her ribs, then down the right side towards the right lower quarter. I wondered whether I could feel a little more resistance than usual as my hand travelled below her navel, but kept it to myself. Whatever was there didn't hurt. I asked Bill to bring her to the surgery the next morning, and left her a small bottle, into which I asked her to put a sample of her stool. It wasn't a pleasant job for her, but I told her as gently as I could that I had to ensure that she wasn't bleeding from her bowel.

The following day I confirmed that even though it did not look dark (moderate amounts of blood turn the stool black) there was a small amount of blood in the sample. I phoned our colorectal specialist clinic for an urgent appointment for her.

That was 30 years ago. Ann did have a malignant tumour in the first part of her large bowel, or colon, close to her appendix. It was ulcerated in the centre, and the bleeding had come from the ulcer. That half of her colon was removed, along with some glands and some adjoining tissues, but the surgeon was able to join up the two ends of the severed bowel, and Ann returned home three weeks later, able to carry on with her life. In those days, we were able to provide plenty of nursing care and help in the home. Bill was a brilliant husband and decided to retire and devote himself to his wife. He let out the farmland to neighbours, and Ann and he planned to travel and enjoy their first holiday for many years.

Ann had received a blood transfusion in the hospital, so came home with a haemoglobin of 12.5 grams per decilitre, high enough for her not to need iron tablets to help replace her loss. She ate well, started to put on weight, looked rosy for the first time in years, and only then realized how ill she had really been feeling before the surgery.

Ann's case is typical of how a slow loss of blood over time can cause anaemia that the patient, and often the doctor or nurse, doesn't suspect. As you will gather from the following case histories, she was one of many who, often understandably, leave things later than they should.

Unfortunately, Ann had left things too late. Two years after her surgery, she became ill again. Despite the initial optimism that 'everything had been removed', some cancer cells must already have spread beyond the operation site. An ultrasound scan showed that she had secondary deposits in her liver, and this time it was impossible to remove the cancer. She had chemotherapy, but it was the start of a downward spiral and she died within six months of the tumour's return.

As I was writing this about Ann I had a vivid image of her face in front of me. She was a great patient and accepted what was in front of her at the time with grace and courage. But today it would almost certainly not have happened in this way. For the last 20 years the balance of medical practice has shifted firmly in favour of prevention of serious illness, rather than waiting for the diagnosis to become obvious before treating it. Today, Ann's anaemia would have been picked up at her annual well-woman clinic appointment, two or three years before her haemoglobin had dropped to 9 grams per decilitre. If she hadn't answered her invitation, she would have been chased up by the practice co-ordinator. Our patients are much more used to being called in for what they see as routine appointments, designed to spot early signs of ill health before they become so serious that people become ill. And we are much more aware of which patients haven't been seen lately, and whom to follow up. There is another bonus: surgery, now much more sophisticated, carries a much higher chance of cure than it did in Ann's day.

The man who was 'as fit as a flea'

Malcolm Bennett is a good example of today's management of blood-loss anaemia. He was in his sixtieth year and had never been seriously ill. In his medical file were a few notes on childhood illness, his vaccinations and his one visit to hospital for treatment of haemorrhoids. He had attended three well-man clinics since his fiftieth birthday, and there had been no problems. On his fifty-ninth birthday he received through the post a small packet, inside which were three sample packs, each containing a small spatula and a plastic bag. The instructions were plain enough: each day for three days he had to dip a spatula into a sample of his stool and place it into the bag. When all three were complete, they had to be sent to Dundee University's team for analysis.

This system was rolled out in Scotland in 2006: since then, everyone in their 50s is asked to cooperate in it. The idea is to catch developing bowel cancers as early as possible, preferably before they start to cause symptoms such as pain or blockage, and before the bleeding from such tumours becomes obvious. Malcolm followed the instructions, sent the sample away and thought no more about it. He considered himself 'as fit as a flea', and was supremely confident that his result would be negative.

His confidence was misplaced. Almost by return of post he received another package. Could he repeat the exercise, this time with a different test, to check on the result? The first had shown blood in all three samples.

Alarmed, Malcolm came to see me. I tried to reassure him that he probably had no need to worry and that nine out of ten causes of blood in the stools were benign – such as the haemorrhoids for which he had previously had treatment. However, I would have been foolish to play down the significance of the result too much. I could not rule out the possibility of bleeding from bowel cancer. I took a finger-prick sample of blood, as much to settle my own concern as to assuage his fear. To my surprise it showed a haemoglobin of 12.2 grams per decilitre. This was a full 2 grams below his last well-man reading of nine months before. I decided to take a larger sample from a vein and sent it off to the lab. A drop of nearly 20 per cent in his haemoglobin over nine months strongly suggested that the bleeding was not a minor or a temporary blip in his health. He was clinically anaemic despite being as fit as a flea, and I now feared for him.

The next week we learned that his reticulocyte count was at 5 per cent: the daily bleeding from his bowel was surely not minor. The second set of samples turned out, as I had no doubt that they would, to contain blood. This 'fit as a flea' man now needed extremely urgent attention.

Malcolm was called in for colonoscopy within days. His tumour, like Ann's, was at the beginning of his large bowel, near his appendix. A CAT scan showed that there was one obvious secondary tumour in his liver. That didn't put his surgeon off. The length of colon containing the cancer was removed, as was the area of liver containing the second tumour. Today's surgeons use techniques to minimize blood loss, so Malcolm didn't require a blood transfusion despite the need for removal of major sections of two vital organs. That would not have been possible in Ann's day.

Four years on, Malcolm remains well. He has had annual scans to rule out further secondaries: there have been none. His liver has recovered and even regrown to compensate for the loss of the lobe containing the tumour. He walks our local hills with his dogs, and blesses the day he sent his samples away. And he is no longer anaemic: his haemoglobin is back to 14.5 grams per decilitre, and his reticulocyte count is less than 1 per cent.

What lesson can we take from Ann's and Malcolm's stories? Ann's 'red flag' – the sign that something serious was going on – was my discovery of her anaemia. If Malcolm had not been asked to send off his stool sample, his anaemia would only have been spotted at his next well-man visit, a year further on, and the red flag may well have been flown too late. In either case, the finding of anaemia absolutely had to be followed up. If it had been assumed that either Ann or Malcolm simply needed iron supplements to deal with a form of iron deficiency (a very common error in the past), their true diagnoses would have been delayed, probably well beyond the time that any cure was possible.

The busy wife and mother

Catherine Swanson has, at 47, brought up three boys who are a credit to her. She holds down a job share, doing alternate weeks of three and two days respectively, in a local government office. She has always worked hard, juggling the responsibilities of a mother with those of the family breadwinner. She hasn't time to be ill or have days off to relax by herself. With her two oldest sons now at university and the youngest in sixth form, she has horrendous expenses and not quite enough income to manage easily. So she doesn't admit to herself that she could be unwell or even under par.

As with Ann Morgan, it wasn't Catherine herself who brought up the subject of her health with me: it was her oldest son, John. Now he is in his second year studying for an engineering degree, he only manages to get home two or three times a year. As with Ann's sister Jean, he had noticed the change in his mum only because they hadn't spent time together for four or five months. His youngest brother, Donald, who was still at home, seeing her every day, wasn't aware that something might be wrong. I had been the boys' doctor since they were born, and John felt confident enough to phone me about his worries.

Catherine's notes showed only that she had had heavy periods in her 20s that had been treated successfully with the contraceptive pill – between her pregnancies, of course. But she hadn't renewed her prescription for around five years: her marriage had failed, and presumably she didn't feel the need to continue with them. I was surprised to see that she hadn't called at the surgery for more than three years.

I asked John to get his mum to make an appointment with me, and she did so the following week. She looked weary and thin. She had put on make-up, so I couldn't see her natural skin colour at a glance, but as she shook my hand I noticed her fingernails. I couldn't tell their natural colour, either, because she had coated them with a light red varnish, but there was a striking sign that I couldn't ignore. The upper surfaces of normal nails are usually either bowed outwards or straight. Catherine's were dimpled, so that they were hollow, like tiny spoons. If I had cared to try it out, with her hands held level, palms down, I could have placed a drop of water on one of her nails and it would have stayed there.

Having such spoon-shaped nails is a classic sign of fairly severe and prolonged anaemia, so I had a few questions to ask her. Her notes provided a way into her history. In her mid 40s she was probably approaching, or even in, her menopause. Was that going well, or had her periods, now that she was no longer taking the pill, reverted to the heavy bleeding episodes of 20 years before?

She burst into tears, which surprised me as it was so unlike her to drop her outward show of a strong, competent and businesslike woman in this way. She told me that she had been struggling with heavy painful bleeding for up to two weeks every month for the previous four years. In fact her menstrual difficulties had been one of the reasons for her marriage break-up: they had interfered too often with the sexual side of her marriage. Her husband had found sex else-where, and she had been too embarrassed and humiliated to reveal this very private side of her life with me, or even with the woman doctor in the practice.

I felt very sad about that: we could have helped her much earlier, and it suggested that our patient–doctor relationship had been lacking. However, I carried on with my questions. Had she done anything herself to ease her menstrual prob-lems? Yes, she said, her mother had suggested that she take iron tablets, as this was the traditional way to boost her ability to replace excessive blood loss.

There is a little logic in that decision. A fundamental element in the centre of the haemoglobin molecule is iron. If we can't replace the actual blood that is lost, we can at least improve our ability to replace it if we replace our body's iron stores. That fact has been the basis of the routine treatment of anaemia with iron-containing medicines since the middle of the nineteenth century. Patent medicines containing iron for 'strengthening the blood' were touted to the public, and their success depended on the fact that they might help people feel better for a while, without actually dealing with the cause of their illness. Of course, replacing the loss of blood with extra iron alone won't do anything to restore the proteins and fats that make up the rest of the red cell constituents, nor will it replace all the ingredients in the plasma that are also lost.

So while Catherine was taking her iron tablets, bought from the local health food store (she hadn't taken the advice of our pharmacist, who would certainly have passed her on to me once he had heard her story), she was gradually becoming more and more anaemic. Iron alone could never be her answer.

We – that is, Catherine and I – needed to know why her menstrual blood loss was so copious, and to try to lessen it. She had always had painful periods and her labours had been difficult. The periods had lessened in the years she had been taking the pill, but she had stopped it because her blood pressure had risen. As her blood pressure had fallen again after she stopped it, she didn't want to try it again. So she had depended simply on painkillers to relieve her discomfort and on iron to 'keep up her blood', as she put it.

It hadn't worked. I explained to her that her fingernails suggested that she might have anaemia, and she admitted that the dimples in them had appeared slowly over the last two years. She had thought that this was just another sign of her approaching menopause.

The finger-prick blood sample showed a haemoglobin of just 8 grams per decilitre, well into the anaemic range, so I took a venous sample to send to the lab. I examined her abdomen, and the only possible slight abnormality was a deep-seated tenderness just above her pelvis. In such a position, it could have come from her bladder or her womb: I couldn't tell which. I therefore added an abdominal ultrasound examination to her list of tests, along with a urine sample, and of course asked her to give a stool sample for testing for blood. We had a long talk about the possibilities, at the end of which I prescribed an iron preparation until we had some answers.

They were not long in coming. The venous blood result was clear. It confirmed the low haemoglobin, normal-sized red cells and a reticulocyte count of nearly 10 per cent, strongly suggesting that her bone marrow was working almost flat out to replace a constant loss of blood. Happily, her stools and urine were clear, which left the heavy periods as the probable cause of her anaemia. The ultrasound result confirmed that she had several large fibroids in her uterus. Fibroids are overgrowths of muscle and fibrous tissue in the wall of the womb that lead to lumpiness in the womb lining. During periods the uneven lining often sheds a lot more blood and tissue than would be lost from a smooth, fibroid-free womb. Fibroids are a very common cause of heavy periods, and often of anaemia.

We arranged for Catherine to see our gynaecological team and she was booked for investigations and surgery later that month. In the meantime she carried on taking the tablets. In the past, she would have had little choice of operation type: she would have had a hysterectomy. Surgical removal of the womb in a total hysterectomy would have solved her bleeding problem permanently, but it has its downsides. Naturally no woman wishes to lose her womb, even when it has caused as much trouble as hers had to Catherine. The operation can have serious effects on a woman's libido and sexual satisfaction – two aspects of such surgery that had not been fully understood until the end of last century.

So every effort is made today to keep the womb in place. Our gynaecologist recommended embolization of her fibroids. This involves passing a catheter (a very fine tube) up an artery in a leg until its tip reaches the branches off to the womb. Specialist scanning techniques then guide the tip into the smaller arteries that feed the fibroids with blood. As each fibroid is usually fed by a single artery, it is possible to pass tiny spheres into it to block it, stopping the blood flow to each fibroid in turn. Over the next few days, the fibroids shrink away, leaving the womb a normal shape and much less likely to bleed excessively when the periods return.

In Catherine's case the embolization was a huge success. Her next period was light and pain-free – the first time, she said, since she was 17. Her iron tablets were stopped, and within three months, without the need for more of them or for a blood transfusion, she had a haemoglobin of 13.5 grams per decilitre, and was therefore no longer anaemic. She continues to have light periods and little discomfort from them.

Our lessons from Catherine?

We assume that, because of their monthly loss of blood, the normal haemoglobin range for women is naturally lower than that for men. In too many women that loss of blood is excessive, leading to even lower levels of haemoglobin. Please, if that describes what you are going through, don't hesitate to get help. Today, we always have some way of correcting the blood loss and the anaemia. It isn't enough, however, just to take medication: we have to establish why the loss is so high, and correct the problem.

This wasn't the only lesson from Catherine's case. Remember those spoon-shaped fingernails? The medical term for this is **koilonychia**. Nails, which are a strong sheet of a fibrous substance called keratin, grow from a layer of basal cells that lie underneath the 'quick'. Iron is a fundamental element within keratin, and if the cells don't have the necessary iron supply the nail that they produce is much softer and thinner than normal. When we use our fingers and thumbs in everyday activities, such as pressing on objects or surfaces, the nail bends with the pressure, so that the upper surface becomes concave rather than convex or straight. Relative lack of iron in the bloodstream is the only cause of this nail shape, so koilonychia is a definitive sign of iron-deficiency anaemia. If you notice your nails changing in this way, you should show them to your doctor. I've had manicurists refer their customers to me purely because they noticed the spoon shape. In each case the patients had felt quite well, had thought nothing of their nail change, and were astonished by their blood test findings.

Hairdressers also have their part to play in referring their customers to us. Keratin is a basic constituent of hair, so hair needs a good supply of iron as much as do nails. In iron deficiency your hair can become thin, brittle and sparse, and grows more slowly. Women naturally notice these changes more than do men, but they hardly ever suspect that iron-deficiency anaemia could be the cause. They tend to go to their hairdresser with the problem rather than coming to us. Yet if we know our patients well, seeing them perhaps only once or twice a year, we notice the hair changes too. When women used to have permanent waves, or perms, one of the signs of iron-deficiency anaemia was that they would stop having them, because the perms made the hair loss more obvious. Now that most women use conditioners, their hair is thicker and less brittle, so it is not so noticeable. When asked outright whether her hair had changed recently, Catherine admitted that it had, but she had put it down to a new shampoo that she thought had dried her hair out. A new conditioner, suggested to her by her hairdresser, seemed to have sorted it. For me, that was another pointer to her anaemia.

Remember, too, that Catherine had made herself up before coming to the surgery. That wasn't a wise move, as I nearly missed yet another of the clues that she might be anaemic. She was wearing bright red lipstick that overlapped her true lip line and smudged the corners of her mouth. Having noted her nails, I asked her to take off her lipstick, which revealed the usual pale lips and cracks, with redness at each corner. Medically this is known as angular stomatitis, and like koilonychia it is a classical sign of longstanding anaemia.

The next step was to see her tongue. Although she hadn't brought up the subject when talking about her symptoms, she now admitted that the angles at the corners of her mouth had been painful, and that her tongue was often uncomfortable. It felt 'burny', she said, even when eating mildly flavoured food. She had always enjoyed spicy food – as a student she had shared a room with an Indian colleague, who had taught her how to cook authentic curries – but recently she had noticed that 'hot' foods hurt her tongue. I asked her to show it to me, and wasn't surprised to see that its surface was smooth and shiny: the little lumps we see on a normal tongue had gone.

Like koilonychia and angular stomatitis, this change in the tongue (atrophic glossitis) was yet another sign that Catherine was severely anaemic, probably due to iron deficiency, and had been so for a long time, perhaps years. Yet she hadn't found the time to come to me about them. She had been 'just too busy'.

The gallstone bleed

Raymond Imrie's anaemia, like Malcolm's, came as a bolt from the blue to him. A haemoglobin of 10.5 grams per decilitre was the only odd finding at his well-man visit. His wife had had to goad him into attending because he felt so fit, and like many other men in their 50s he didn't have the time to spare.

That reading was a red flag to his doctor, who took the time to ask a series of questions. Did he have any health problems? No. Was his weight steady? How was his appetite? Fine. Did he have any problems with his bowels or urine? No. Had he noticed any bleeding? No. Did he ever experience pain? No. Well, maybe on odd occasions a little indigestion after food. Always just below his ribs, on the right side. But it was so rare that he didn't bother with it.

His doctor didn't think much of that symptom, either, but felt it was the only possible pointer to a cause. Raymond responded normally to an abdominal examination, but that wasn't the end of his doctor's interest. A full blood count showed a rise in Raymond's reticulocytes, and red cells that were much smaller than normal. Instead of his red cells having an average volume of around 85 cubic micrometres (see Table 1 on p. 3), the reading was in the 60s. This was a strong indication of bleeding from somewhere. It showed up in his stools: as with Malcolm's case, it wasn't enough to be seen with the naked eye, but it was there in each of three consecutive samples.

Raymond's next visit was to the gastroenterologist, who found that his 'little indigestion' was not so little after all. An ultrasound scan showed that he had a single gallstone stuck in the tube (the common bile duct) between his gall bladder and his duodenum (the first part of the small bowel). An endoscopy (a flexible fibre-optic tube examination passed down the throat into the stomach and duodenum) showed that it had eroded the duct wall, causing a chronic ulcer. The blood was oozing from that site. It only needed a few millilitres of loss every day to cause his chronic anaemia.

That endoscopy led to his cure, as well as his diagnosis. Using the fibre-optic technology, the gastroenterologist was able to crush the stone and flush its remains away into the bowel. Raymond's bleeding was cured at a one-step visit to the hospital. The duct healed and his haemoglobin started to climb. Without the need for treatment, his haemoglobin climbed back into the normal range within three months.

Raymond was lucky that it had been dealt with so quickly and easily. That gallstone might have eroded completely through the duct wall, leading to leakage of bile into the abdominal cavity – causing biliary peritonitis, a very serious, even life-threatening condition that would have led to emergency surgery and a much longer and more distressing stay in hospital.

His case is admittedly unusual, less common than the others, but I've included it as an example of a cause of anaemia that might in earlier times have been diagnosed as an iron-deficiency anaemia and treated with iron supplements and advice on eating more healthily. After all, he had no symptoms to speak of, was feeling well and did not appear ill. He would have been a classic case of 'poor iron-absorption anaemia' and treated accordingly. That mistake could have been fatal for him. Happily, today's doctors are far more aware than their predecessors of the dangers of coming to such conclusions.

Learning lessons from cases

You will have gathered from reading this chapter that it isn't enough to accept that anaemia is a consequence of 'iron deficiency' and that replacing that missing iron is a satisfactory treatment for it. We absolutely must try to find the cause of the anaemia and correct it. However, there are times when taking iron is at least part of the answer. Iron-deficiency anaemia may be the result of many illnesses, and replacing the iron is often an important part of the cure. It is very rarely, however, the whole cure. The next chapter explains why.

3

Why we need iron

The role of iron in our bodies is crucial to our understanding of why anaemia is so common. I've written about the red pigment of haemoglobin, which combines so easily with oxygen in our lungs and carries it around the bloodstream to deliver it to our organs and tissues. At the heart of each haemoglobin molecule is an iron atom. Without it, haemoglobin can't form and we couldn't pick up the oxygen we need to live. The process can be explained as simply as that. If we don't deliver enough iron to our bone marrow, where our red cells are made, then we are bound to become anaemic.

After we are born, our only source of iron is our food. However, the process of building up iron reserves (in our liver) starts when we are in our mother's womb. Developing babies are highly efficient in extracting iron from their mother's blood through the placenta (afterbirth). They store much of the iron in their liver, and the rest of it goes to their bone marrow, where it is processed into haemoglobin and red blood cells. Babies' livers have a plentiful iron store, and they usually have more than enough haemoglobin to serve their oxygen needs for the first few months of life. The placenta is so efficient at sucking iron from the mother's bloodstream into the baby's circulation that it is extremely rare for babies to be anaemic at birth: their mothers have to be very anaemic in the first place for this to occur. I've written more about anaemia in pregnancy in a later chapter.

Once we are born, however, obtaining enough iron to keep up our haemoglobin levels is a much more difficult matter.

For the first few months after birth our still immature digestive system finds it very hard to take up enough iron from our mother's milk to maintain our red cell production. We start off life with a high haemoglobin, thanks to Mum, but over the first two months it drops from around 16 to 17 grams per decilitre to between 11 and 12 grams per decilitre. Our ability to digest iron improves as our gut systems begin to mature, so that our haemoglobin level rises steadily throughout our first decade to 12.5 grams per decilitre. It doesn't reach the adult norm of around 14 grams per decilitre until we are 14 years old. During these early years of very fast growth, our bone marrow is constantly working flat out to increase our red cell numbers enormously, just to keep up with the ever-escalating demand. This process continues through teenage years, making further demands on our bone marrow and on our iron stores, just to keep our red cell production in a range that will avoid severe anaemia.

In the vast majority of children the bone marrow seems to manage well enough, but a few children can become anaemic simply from not being able to maintain red cell production. This form of childhood anaemia, due exclusively to poor nutrition, has been almost eradicated in the Global North, being limited to socially very deprived families (or the occasional very food-faddy family) whose eating habits don't give them enough iron-containing foods. From the early teens onwards, however, it can show itself for the first time. Girls – even girls who eat well – are much more likely than boys to become anaemic as they enter puberty, when their fast growth spurt combined with the start of monthly bleeding puts even greater strain on their iron stores. Many girls become iron-deficient without their parents suspecting it: they see tiredness and lack of energy as just the usual behaviour of an adolescent girl, when they are the cardinal signs of moderately severe anaemia.

Unfortunately, anaemia isn't the only outcome of being iron-deficient in early life. Iron deficiency has been linked with poor physical and intellectual development. As long ago as 1991, a study showed that babies found to have iron-deficiency anaemia in infancy, despite its being corrected very early, scored lower on mental and physical tests when they were five years old than children of the same age who had not been anaemic (Lozoff et al. 1991). Other researchers have confirmed these results, so paediatricians take iron-deficiency anaemia in childhood very seriously. However, its cure is rarely just a matter of giving the child extra iron in the form of medicines. Iron deficiency in such children strongly indicates that their whole home environment and their families' eating habits have to be reviewed and corrected, where possible. Anaemia in children with normally formed red cells (children with inherited abnormalities in their red cells are covered later) is almost always the result of extremely poor general nutrition. Iron supplements may help, but better eating is crucial. It must be managed completely, with tactful but firm parental guidance into better eating for the whole family.

Why should iron deficiency be such a worry, when iron itself is one of the commonest elements? The reason is simply that our digestive system can't absorb more than a tiny amount of iron – as little as 1 milligram (mg) – from our food in a day. That is only just enough to balance our daily loss of a milligram or so from shed scales of skin and lining cells from our intestines. Red cells last for around three months, and when they break down, releasing their iron into the circulation, the liver is extremely efficient at capturing it and returning it to the bone marrow. So as long as there is no abnormal bleeding, our bodies need very little extra iron from our food. However, if we start to lose blood we find it very difficult to replace the iron lost.

For women this need for iron can easily become a crisis, because they lose around 20 to 40 mg a month in their monthly menstruation: they make it up by doubling their ability to absorb iron from their food to 2 mg per day. When adults of either gender become anaemic they can raise their daily iron absorption to a maximum of around 6 mg per day, but that usually only manages to balance, and not overcome, their daily loss of iron from their underlying condition. My patient histories in Chapter 2 are graphic examples of this.

Taking in more iron than we can absorb simply means that we excrete it in our stools: that is why our motions turn black when we swallow a daily iron tablet. The excess iron (each pill contains at least 50 mg of iron, more than eight times the maximum we can absorb) simply runs through our stomach, small intestine and large bowel without being absorbed. So once we are anaemic, iron replacement in pills and medicines helps but is rarely the sole answer. We need to follow the message that runs through this book: that cure lies in finding the cause of the iron loss and correcting it.

However, people who are found to be anaemic need treatment while the cause is being sought. So doctors *do* prescribe iron tablets, capsules or medicines in the meantime, to boost the supply of iron to the bone marrow, and to build up the depleted iron stores in the liver. If you are anaemic, therefore, you should be familiar with the pros and cons of the current iron prescriptions. Before doing so, I repeat the warning that you shouldn't be buying iron treatments from shops without knowing for sure that you are anaemic, that the cause is known, that the correct treatment is iron replacement, and that the type you choose is approved by your doctor. If you are treating yourself, you must let your doctor know you are doing so.

Iron treatments in anaemia

The accepted theories on the most effective way to use iron when treating anaemia differ widely, depending on whether you are an expert in the United Kingdom or in the United States. Being a British doctor working wholly in the National Health Service, I'm happy to stick with the British guidelines, but I have added the opinions of two distinguished US physicians, Drs Kenneth Bridges and Howard A. Pearson, to offer you balance.

The British view

Here I'm drawing from the *British National Formulary* (*BNF*), the quarterly handbook sent to all British prescribing doctors. We use it as our standard when considering prescribing for our patients: it is written by groups of specialists known for their excellence in their fields, and updated several times a year.

The introduction to the section on iron-deficiency anaemias stresses that treating patients with an iron preparation is justified only when there is demonstrable iron deficiency, and that before starting treatment the doctor must exclude any serious underlying cause of the anaemia. It adds that prevention of anaemia with an iron preparation is appropriate in 'malabsorption, menorrhagia, pregnancy, after operations to remove the stomach (gastrectomy), in patients on haemodialysis, and in low-weight newborn babies'. I've mentioned the babies already, and will cover all these other conditions in later chapters.

So once the underlying cause has been found, it is correct to give people with anaemia iron – but with which type of medicine, and with which iron compound? This is where the Brits and Yanks differ.

Our *BNF* is clear where it stands. Iron should be given

by mouth, it says, unless there are good reasons for using another route (such as injections into muscle or vein). The choice of iron-containing pills is wide, but they don't differ much in the amount of iron each delivers into our circulation, so the choice depends on cost and on how well each individual can tolerate them. The cheapest and commonest of them is ferrous sulphate.

Ferrous sulphate tablets have the reputation of making people feel sick and causing indigestion (mainly upper stomach pains). They make some people constipated and others have diarrhoea, so it's difficult to predict beforehand which side effect they may have on you, if any. According to the *BNF*, when the different iron compounds are compared in well-conducted trials, ferrous sulphate is no worse than any other in causing side effects. Much depends on how much iron is in the drug dose. It is suggested that if you do have side effects from ferrous sulphate, it's better first to reduce the dose rather than to switch to another preparation, the two main ones being ferrous gluconate and ferrous fumarate.

I'm not sure that this advice is appropriate for everyone needing iron pills. In practice I've occasionally had to ring the changes from the sulphate to either the gluconate or the fumarate. Some people find that one of them is more acceptable than the others, and are happy with the outcome. The choice seems to depend on feeling comfortable in the time shortly after swallowing it, and on whether or not the tablets make you constipated. There are also two iron-containing elixirs. One is a polysaccharide-iron complex (Niferex) and the other is sodium iron edetate (Sytron). They are used mainly for babies and children, and for the very few adults who can't swallow pills.

Some iron preparations contain vitamin C, on the grounds that this may help the iron to be absorbed more efficiently: the *BNF* states that the advantage is 'minimal' and not worth the extra cost. It also does not recommend taking slow-release iron capsules or tablets. Although they are more convenient as a once-daily tablet (the others are taken twice a day), the gradual release of iron over hours means that most of the iron isn't available for absorption until the tablets reach the lower part of the bowel, in which iron uptake is very small. We take up most of our iron in the duodenum, the upper part of the small intestine close to the stomach, so that slow release can miss the point of the medication.

The US viewpoint on iron

It is odd that the two nations' experts can differ so widely in their take on something as apparently simple as iron tablets. Drs Bridges and Pearson write that ferrous sulphate is 'tolerated poorly' by many people because it causes cramps, bloating or constipation, and that it is the sulphate part of the molecule that produces these. They add that ferrous gluconate is a good alternative, and is cheaper than the equally innocuous ferrous fumarate. They promote the polysaccharide-iron complex for adults as well as children as being better tolerated than the other preparations, but admit that its higher cost is a disadvantage. Curiously, they also admit that there is no information on how well iron is absorbed from it.

Drs Bridges and Pearson mention a form of metallic iron, not in chemical combination, that is delivered to the bowel wall in the form of a 'macromolecular complex' of tiny spheres only 2 micrometres across. Called carbonyl iron, it is referred to as being non-toxic and exceptionally well tolerated. It is not available yet in the United Kingdom.

Where the US doctors most disagree with the Brits is on the addition of vitamin C to iron tablets. They say that the vitamin 'substantially boosts iron absorption', especially when the two are combined last thing at night. The gut slows down during sleep, so the combination has two advantages over the usual daily tablet: the iron stays longer in contact with the vital upper part of the bowel, and the vitamin C promotes its absorption. However, they don't approve of their patients swallowing tablets that combine the iron and the vitamin in one dose. Instead they suggest that, along with the iron tablet, people take a vitamin C tablet in orange juice. They say that this costs much less than the combined tablet.

However, the final choice for the US doctors, and in their opinion the most effective way to correct iron-deficiency anaemia, is to eat red meat. Haem (the active part of the haemoglobin molecule) is the most readily absorbed form of iron, and its main source is meat. Iron uptake from haem is not limited by the mechanisms that limit the uptake from iron-containing pills. They ruefully conclude, however, that 'meat often is not an option due sometimes to dietary preferences and at other times to limited finances'.

Making sense of the debate

Where do I stand in this transatlantic debate? I'm with the Brits on most of it. My experience as a family doctor leads me to conclude that most people are easily able to tolerate one of the three standard iron pills listed in the *BNF*, and don't mind taking one of them twice a day. It is exceptional for people to have to change to one of the more expensive, more complicated and not necessarily more effective iron preparations. However, these are always available as a backstop when someone really can't take the usual forms of iron. I quite like the thought that patients might take orange juice with an iron tablet before bedtime, though I wouldn't prescribe vitamin C tablets with it. I accept that adding vitamin C will make little difference to the amount of iron that a patient can absorb. Remember that we can only absorb a maximum of 6 mg iron a day, and that every iron tablet contains more than 50 mg, some of them much more. So on any form of iron treatment, we excrete far more of the iron than we could possibly absorb. After all, the aim of the treatment isn't primarily to improve our daily absorption of iron, but to cure the anaemia. What we need to see in our patients on any of these forms of iron is their haemoglobin levels increasing every month up to normal levels.

Whichever tablet we use, we aim to increase your haemoglobin level by around 2 grams per decilitre every three to four weeks. We cannot expect a faster rise in blood levels because you cannot absorb enough iron every day, even on maximum doses of iron, to make the recovery faster. So a person starting with a haemoglobin of 8 grams per decilitre can expect it to take three months to return to a normal, non-anaemic haemoglobin level.

When your haemoglobin eventually rises into the normal range (from 13.5 grams per decilitre for women and from 14.5 grams per decilitre for men), we still continue to prescribe iron for you for at least another three months, so as to build up iron stores in your liver. After that, the iron treatment is stopped, and we monitor your blood for up to a year afterwards to check that you are not falling back into anaemia with a dropping haemoglobin level.

Interestingly, very soon after you start treatment, even before there is a significant rise in your haemoglobin (here I have assumed that the cause of your anaemia has been found and corrected), you will start to feel much better. This is difficult to explain: there must be more to feeling unwell when you are anaemic than simply a fall in your red cell count or your haemoglobin. We don't know why this is: it is difficult, if not impossible, to correlate grades of feeling well with any measurable physical test result.

What if I don't respond to iron treatment?

So you have started on iron treatment, but a month later your haemoglobin has stayed stubbornly at an anaemic level and has not risen. What next? Please forgive your doctor if he or she asks if you are actually taking your tablets as advised, as not doing so is the commonest cause of lack of response. That isn't surprising, as discomfort after taking iron is relatively common, and it is natural not to want to continue the treatment. Understandably, people tend to be too embarrassed to admit to their doctors that they haven't been following advice: often we have to ask pointed questions before they own up. When they do, it is usually simple to find another type of iron pill that is less likely to cause problems. We won't blame you or think any the less of you if that's what you have done, so please don't feel guilty about it.

However, if you have been taking the tablets and have still not responded, we must look for other reasons for the treatment failure. There are plenty of them. The crucial one is that you may still be bleeding internally (usually from the stomach or bowel – see the case histories in Chapter 2) without knowing it, and the bleeding is causing you to lose more blood than your iron treatment can replace. Naturally, your doctor will need to repeat all the tests you had in the beginning to rule that out. If they turn out to be negative, then something is stopping the iron from being absorbed. That something may be a surprise to you: it may be nothing more than the fact that you are taking other prescription drugs that interfere with your iron uptake, or that you enjoy a good strong cup of tea.

Anti-ulcer drugs

For more than 30 years we have had marvellous medicines for treating duodenal and stomach ulcers caused mostly by the acidity of the digestive juices produced by our stomach. Before the medicines were developed, we had to remove the seven-eighths of the stomach surface that produced the acid in order to cure chronic ulcer problems. Gastrectomy – surgical removal of most of the stomach – was the commonest operation. There was at least one on every surgeon's list.

Today's doctors have never watched or performed a gastrectomy for ulcers. The drugs that replaced it, designed to minimize levels of stomach acid or eliminate it altogether, have been so successful that they are household names. Tagamet (cimetidine), Zantac (ranitidine), Losec (omeprazole) and Zoton (lansoprazole) are among them. However, to absorb enough iron to correct anaemia, we need some stomach acid: without it, we can't absorb enough to replace the lost iron stores in the liver. So if you are taking one of these acid-reducing or acid-eliminating drugs along with iron, you need to separate the two medication times as widely as possible. It is a common combination, because excessive stomach acidity often leads to bleeding from the stomach wall and therefore to anaemia.

Faced with a person with anaemia who needs to stay on anti-ulcer drugs and also to take iron, most family doctors would advise you to take the iron first thing in the morning on an empty stomach, and to wait for an hour before taking the ulcer treatment. That way, 23 hours after the last dose, you should have enough acid to digest the iron and still protect your stomach.

Tea and coffee

Tea seems, and actually is, an innocuous beverage. It tastes pleasant, makes you feel good, and has substances in it, like theobromine, caffeine and theophylline, that give you a kick. Before we had modern medicines for asthma, doctors prescribed tea because the 'theo' chemicals opened up the bronchial tubes, helping people to breathe more deeply and curing wheeze. But tea, especially black strong tea, also contains tannins, which bond very strongly with iron to form complexes that we can't absorb. The result? The iron simply passes all the way through your digestive system, and you remain anaemic. It is sometimes really difficult to get even that tiny amount of 1 to 6 mg of iron a day into your circulation!

Sometimes the answer is simply to take your iron tablets on an empty stomach, with a little water if you need to, and not to drink tea within an hour of doing so. If you drink tea with a meal, its effect on iron absorption lasts even longer, so when you are taking iron tablets and must have your cup of tea, make sure that you drink it at least an hour after your last mouthful of food, and that you take your iron tablet preferably more than half an hour before the meal, quite separately from your cup that cheers.

What about coffee as an alternative? You need to be warned about that too. Coffee, like tea, combines strongly with iron salts, but in this case the body can absorb the combination. That isn't much good either, however, because once in the circulation the coffee–iron combination stays bonded together, so that we can't use the iron. Even more important is that coffee-drinking new mothers pass the combination on in their breast milk, with the result that the nursing baby doesn't get the advantage of the iron and can become anaemic. So pregnant and nursing mothers who need iron tablets should go easy on their coffee habit, only drinking it in small amounts at times well separated from their iron tablets.

There is an extra point about feeding babies that needs emphasizing. Mothers who have had to give up breast feeding early, for whatever reason, should be aware that cow's milk, although it contains around the same amount of iron as breast milk, can sometimes irritate a small baby's duodenal lining. As with adults, babies absorb iron in milk through the duodenum, so those fed almost exclusively on cow's milk can become iron-deficient and anaemic, because of the irritation it may cause. Iron supplements aren't effective unless Mum can switch to another source of milk that isn't irritant. Expressed human milk is the best option, but that is obviously not an answer for most parents. If you have any doubts that your baby isn't doing as well on your alternative to breast milk as he or she should, talk to your doctor about the possibility of anaemia.

This said about tea and coffee, I must add that I haven't ever come across a case of an anaemic adult failing to respond to iron simply because of an addiction to either drink. There are other causes, apart from the common one of continuing blood loss from the bowel that was covered in Chapter 2, that may only come to light because a person has failed to respond with a rise in haemoglobin to the first month of iron treatment.

One, for example, is that despite swallowing the iron tablets exactly as instructed, you just can't absorb it. Eileen Lloyd's case is a good example of this.

Eileen's story – the 'hidden' coeliac

Eileen is a woman of 43 who has crashed through the chief-executive glass ceiling to make a great success of an engineering business. She is well aware that her appearance must be immaculate, and has carefully watched what she eats and how she exercises all her adult life. So it was quite a surprise to me when she visited the surgery looking a little thinner than I remembered her. Her only previous appointments had been for vaccinations against various tropical fevers before business trips to Africa and Central America. I had never known her to be unwell.

Her main complaint was an even bigger surprise. Two or three months before, she had choked, only for a few minutes, when eating a meal. She at first thought that something had gone down the wrong way and dismissed it as a minor and temporary incident. However, the choking came back, and she was now finding it difficult to swallow at some time during most meals. Something seemed to be 'sticking' just below the back of her throat. As an aside, she said that her nails seemed to have changed in the last year or so. She didn't know whether that signified anything but she thought she should mention it.

I looked at her nails. Koilonychia. Iron-deficiency anaemia. The questions started. Had she noticed any blood in her stools or urine? Did she have any digestive discomfort, such as pain or bloating? Were her periods very heavy? Was she taking aspirin or any medication that might have caused her stomach to bleed? She answered no to all of these questions. Nevertheless, I examined her, and could find nothing abnormal. Her blood test showed that her haemoglobin was only 7.1 grams per decilitre, an astonishingly low figure for someone who appeared to be so well. The blood film under the microscope showed that her red cells were much smaller than normal and were pale in the middle – there was only a rim of red around their outer margins.

The report also commented that the platelet count (platelets are tiny fragments of cells that are involved in blood clotting) was extremely high – well above the normal limit. The haematologist confirmed that this was typical of a longstanding and severe iron-deficiency anaemia. How could this have come about, when to all outward appearances she was living a perfectly normal healthy life? Could her diet be a possible cause?

We went into her eating habits together. Conscious about her need to keep slim, she had been eating very little and kept to an almost vegetarian diet. She rarely ate red meat, choosing fish and salads as her usual main meals when dining out, and confining her meals at home to vegetarian dishes. That didn't seem extreme enough to cause anaemia, but I supposed that it was possible.

I asked one of our local hospital physicians to see her urgently, and he quickly confirmed that she wasn't bleeding from the bowel or into her urine, but that her blood picture certainly confirmed that she had a severe iron deficiency. The choking was caused by a 'web' of tissue that had grown across part of her throat near her larynx, narrowing her oesophagus. The diagnosis was made of Plummer-Vinson syndrome.

I remembered Plummer-Vinson syndrome from my student days in Birmingham. If I had been a student in Glasgow it would have been called Paterson-Brown-Kelly syndrome. The universities still argue about which group of doctors described it first. Whatever it should be called, I hadn't seen anyone with it since then. For some people, as was the case for Eileen Lloyd, the only outward sign that they have anaemia is their difficulty with swallowing because of the web that has grown in the throat near their voice-box. They are totally unaware that they are also anaemic.

Because we could find no cause for Eileen's anaemia, and because she had admitted both to me and to her consultant that she ate very little, we felt that she was one of those rare people whose anaemia was probably dietary. Once she started to eat more healthily, and was helped by iron tablets, we predicted that she would gain haemoglobin quickly. After the ENT surgeon gently teased the web away from her throat, under anaesthetic, we thought that she would quickly start to swallow normally again, begin to gain weight and have a haemoglobin of around 9 grams per decilitre when we saw her a month later. We were optimistic that we had solved her problems.

We were wrong. Despite her best efforts at eating more meat and cereals, she didn't improve. In fact she felt worse.

Although the swallowing problem was solved, an hour or so after each of these new meals she developed pains in her upper abdomen, with bloating, and her motions became looser than before. After three weeks she was back in the surgery, feeling ill. Her haemoglobin was still at 7 grams per decilitre.

At last the penny dropped. Looking back on the time, some years before, when she had started on her meagre diet, she remembered that she had made the decision not just because she wanted to keep trim, but because many of the foods that she had given up had tended to make her feel nauseated or gave her loose motions. Returning to them in the last three weeks had brought back unpleasant memories.

This time, on examining her abdomen I found it to be swollen and tender. I was fairly sure that she had adult-onset coeliac disease: her problem was not caused by her eating too little, but by her gut wall reacting badly to foods containing gluten – mainly flour and cereals. Coeliac disease upsets the delicate mechanism for iron absorption in the duodenum, so she couldn't benefit from iron-containing medicines. The consultant performed the relevant tests for coeliac disease, and confirmed the diagnosis.

Everyone has heard of people who react badly to gluten. Supermarkets stock gluten-free foods, and good restaurants will cater to people with gluten sensitivity. But if you don't have a sufferer in your family or as a friend, you probably don't know about the different ways in which it can show itself and the great difficulty that coeliacs have in avoiding gluten completely. Although it is easy to list the foods to avoid, gluten is used as a bulking agent in many manufactured products – such as white pepper – and even the tiny amount swallowed by shaking a pepperpot over a meal is enough to affect the gut. Manufacturers are more careful about labelling their products, but some still slip through the net. And restaurants may not be as assiduous as they should be in giving their customers complete information about gluten content on their menu.

The cause of coeliac disease was discovered by chance in 1945, in the Netherlands during the last few months of the Second World War. These were horrendous times for the Dutch, who starved as almost all their food was confiscated and sent to Germany. In one children's hospital, however, a miracle was happening. A small group of children who up to that time had been very severely anaemic, undernourished and underdeveloped, physically and mentally, suddenly started to grow and become well. Their doctors were sharp enough to link their wonderful progress with the fact that their food was limited to vegetables and occasional fish, and that they no longer had access to foods based on flour or cereals. Gluten in the flour was identified as the substance that had been wreaking havoc in the children's digestive systems and holding them back.

Since then, the first diagnosis we think of in children who are not thriving, who have constant stomach pains and pass bulky, apparently semi-digested stools, is coeliac disease. By the time they are two years old, almost all of them are on their lifelong gluten-free diet, and they do very well. They are warned as they grow older that if they lapse they will become ill again: very few of them do. This is the picture that most of us have of coeliac disease.

However, there is an adult-onset form of the illness. People who have eaten normally throughout their childhood may not start to have symptoms until their 20s or 30s. Because these symptoms are difficult to define – tummy pains, bloating, wind, loose motions are the common ones – they are easily confused with dietary indiscretions or irritable bowel. Sometimes, as with Eileen, people don't seek their doctor's help for them, preferring to stick to over-the-counter indigestion remedies. It may be years before they eventually do so, by which time they are often seriously anaemic. In Eileen's case, her main complaint, her choking, was unrelated to her coeliac disease. The web was the direct result of her low haemoglobin – it only forms when people have been seriously iron-deficient.

Why had she become anaemic? In coeliac disease, the lining cells of the duodenum, the area of the gut in which most iron is absorbed, react with an inflammatory response to the gluten. The result is that their ability to absorb the iron (among other nutrients) is lost, and over months the person becomes iron-deficient. The bone marrow can continue to take iron from the stores in the liver, but anaemia becomes inevitable. As the process is slow, the patient may not even notice the day-to-day deterioration.

Eileen's case is unusual in that as her iron deficiency worsened she developed Plummer-Vinson syndrome, and this was the stimulus that brought her to the doctor. In a sense she was lucky that it did so, because many people with adult coeliac disease continue to struggle on until they are even more anaemic than she was.

What did I learn from Eileen's case? Primarily, that I won't assume again that anaemia is due to a faddy diet without first ruling out everything else. Looking back on her case, I suppose that she would have been a typical case of nutritional anaemia and that we couldn't be blamed for our mistaken assumption. However, in future I will keep coeliac disease in mind when faced with an adult with anaemia of unknown cause.

Eileen's management

Once we knew the cause of Eileen's anaemia, we initiated her into the intricacies of managing life as an adult with coeliac disease. It means avoiding every trace of gluten in her food.

She has to be meticulous in learning all the foods, sauces and condiments that might contain gluten, and how to avoid eating them even accidentally. She has learned to be tactful when out for dinner, and to prepare much more of her own food for herself rather than taking the easy way out with the odd ready meal. She has joined Coeliac UK, <www.coeliac. org.uk>, which she has found useful in providing masses of facts about how to manage the condition as well as possible.

Once started on a gluten-free eating pattern – we hesitate to call it a diet as her new habits have to be lifelong – Eileen felt well within days. She did continue on iron tablets along with her food, and had no digestive problems with them. A month later her haemoglobin was 9.5 grams per decilitre; a year later it was 15. We counted her management as a great success, with one chastening proviso.

Although we do not expect the web in her throat to return, we know from histories of past cases of Plummer-Vinson syndrome that it is linked to the development of oesophageal cancer, so Eileen has had to be put on regular endoscopy follow-up to ensure that any changes towards a tumour development are identified in time.

Eileen sees this as a minor inconvenience and is grateful that she has been given a new lease of life. Her iron treatment was stopped after three months, and we are confident that she will have a normal future without anaemia.

Iron – a poison?

Colin's story

I can't leave this chapter about iron without a warning. Iron tablets in the wrong hands can be a poison, and the results can be lethal. I met Colin more than 40 years ago, but at times I still see in my mind's eye his agonized face and his small tortured body. He was two years old, and like any normal two-year-old he was into everything he could get his hands on. Unhappily, what he had got his hands on were his mother's iron tablets. They were attractively presented in see-through clear capsules, and the tiny coloured spheres inside them looked just like the hundreds and thousands in any sweet shop or supermarket.

Mum had left her handbag open, and he had seen them and had wolfed down four or five before she saw him and put them away out of reach. What should she do? They were only iron tablets, after all, she reasoned, and surely couldn't do any harm. It was three in the afternoon, her husband would soon be home from work and she had a younger baby to deal with. So she adopted a 'wait and see' approach, and sat Colin down to play with his toys. It was nearly a fatal decision.

By four o'clock Colin was complaining of a really sore tummy. He was crying and vomiting, and the vomit looked like coffee grounds. He was 'seeing things' and extremely distressed. His mum finally took the right course of action. She called an ambulance, said that the problem might be caused by his taking her iron tablets, and he was in our Accident and Emergency Department within the next 15 minutes.

I was the house officer on duty: by the time Colin had reached us, he was drowsy and floppy, hardly able to respond to our very gentle questioning. While we were taking blood samples from him (he hardly noticed the needle) our consultant paediatrician had organized an intravenous injection of desferrioxamine, a chemical that would 'bind' the excess iron that had reached his bloodstream and reduce the massive amounts of iron that were poisoning his brain and liver.

After several anxious hours Colin started to recover, and within another two days he was fit to go home. But it was touch and go for a while. Overdoses of iron pills, almost always taken by accident by a child aged between two and four, can kill. Untreated, after a few hours they go into shock, fall into a coma and die from acute liver failure. Sometimes the diagnosis is missed because the parents have not noticed that the pills are missing. The tragedy is then compounded hugely by their unending sense of guilt at leaving their child in such danger.

Children can only tolerate very small quantities of iron, and even a few of their parents' tablets will swamp their liver with the metal and lead to acute liver failure. We have to remove the iron from the body as fast as possible, and that is done by a chelating agent – one that 'collects' the iron – such as desferrioxamine.

The lesson from Colin's case? If you are taking any form of iron you absolutely *must* keep the tablets in a safe place, well away from where any child can see or reach them. It doesn't matter if there is no child in your house. Most people have children visiting from time to time, and visiting children can be as curious and fearless as a child of your own. This applies very much to grandparents (many of whom take iron), as well as to people whose friends and other family are visiting.

This last warning may seem over the top, but it isn't. I have known two children who swallowed iron tablets when visiting other homes, one of whom tragically died. It took only seconds, while the hostess was out of the room. The tablets were beside a lounge chair, in a supposedly childproof bottle, the lid of which was left loose because the lady, with arthritic fingers, had found it difficult to open. It's normal to keep your medicines in a safe cupboard, out of sight, but people often see iron as a mineral supplement and not really a 'medicine', so they don't take the same care of it as they would their other prescription medicines. That attitude can be a terrible mistake.

You will have gathered by now that absorbing iron from our food can be a tricky business, and that if our digestive system is disturbed, our iron uptake rate is one of the first essentials to be lost. I used coeliac disease as an example of a direct effect of a disorder of the gut that leads to iron-deficient anaemia. However, there are several general illnesses not primarily affecting the gut that can also cause us to become anaemic. They are the subject of Chapters 5 and beyond.

Chapter 4 is the one I promised you about pregnancy. Pregnancy, of course, isn't an illness but a wonderfully natural condition that happens to almost half of the human race and at the same time profoundly affects the other half. For many years, the first advice that every woman was given when attending her doctor and midwife for her initial antenatal visit was that she had to take an iron tablet every day. Was that advice correct? Did it mean that every pregnant woman was relatively anaemic? Was it the unnecessary medicalization of a natural state? These are the questions discussed in Chapter 4.

4

Anaemia in pregnancy

If you are a woman who had her children in the era from the 1950s to the 1990s, you will remember that at your first visit to your doctor about your pregnancy, probably after missing two periods, you were given a prescription for a combination of iron and folic acid. You were asked to take it before you knew the result of your blood test, and to continue it throughout the pregnancy, regardless of the result. It was assumed that extra iron would keep your haemoglobin levels high, for your sake and your baby's. It was also assumed that every pregnant woman became relatively anaemic in comparison with her previously non-anaemic, non-pregnant state, and that iron tablets could only do good and never harm.

Today that attitude is looked on as out of date, although some doctors still find it hard to abandon. We only give iron tablets if blood tests reveal true anaemia, and we follow up every woman throughout the pregnancy to make sure we don't miss it. Why have we changed? We have a better understanding of how pregnancy changes a woman's circulation, and we recognize that it is normal for her haemoglobin to fall to what would in non-pregnant women be classified as anaemic levels. We would not give her iron unless the fall was much greater than this norm.

What happens during pregnancy to make this change in haemoglobin? Her fast-growing womb, her placenta and her developing foetus produce considerable changes in the woman's circulation. The biggest one is that the volume of the circulating plasma, the clear fluid in which the red cells float, increases. It starts to rise in the sixth week after conception. By the middle of the pregnancy the circulation is 30 per cent larger in volume than before, and by the baby's birth it is 50 per cent higher. The heart is pushing round the body a total blood volume that is half as much again as the pre-pregnant circulation.

During the same period the number of red cells and the total haemoglobin (the amount of haemoglobin in all of the blood) each rise by between 20 and 30 per cent. So during pregnancy, women increase their oxygen-carrying power (as shown by the total haemoglobin) by 20 to 30 per cent. As the true measure of anaemia is how much oxygen-carrying power is in the circulation, the extra carrying power of the increase in haemoglobin and red cells is more than enough to ensure that the mother is far from anaemic and the baby is getting plenty of oxygen through the placenta.

However, standard blood tests, such as red cell counts and haemoglobin levels, don't give that impression. Because the total volume of the plasma has increased by much more than the volume of red cells, the haematocrit (the proportion of red cells to plasma) inevitably falls. (Remember the haematocrit in Table 1 on p. 3.) Instead of the red cells accounting for 45 per cent of the total blood volume, they now show as only 35 to 40 per cent. And the numbers of red cells in the test sample have fallen too, from around 5 million per microlitre to 4 million, even though there are more than enough to ensure good oxygen for both mother and baby.

The result of these changes is that haemoglobin levels that we used to think showed anaemia in pregnancy are in fact normal. They start at an average of 12.5 grams per decilitre at four weeks, fall to 11.8 at ten weeks, then to 11.2 from the fifteenth to the thirtieth weeks, rising back to 12 only at the fortieth week, at full term (Bridges and Pearson 2008, p. 47). How can this be an advantage for the baby? Experts in blood flow point out that with the reduced red cell volume, the blood flows much more smoothly: it is less viscous, or sticky, and this allows much smoother and faster flow through the placenta, so that the entry of nutritious substances, alongside oxygen, and the exit of waste products can be much more efficient than if the haematocrit were higher. In the past, a haemoglobin reading of 11 grams per decilitre would have been taken as a sign of anaemia: now, in mid-pregnancy it is considered normal.

So does this mean that we no longer need to give pregnant women iron? If they have enough haemoglobin to service the needs of both their babies and themselves, why should they have to take pills? In order to 'build' a baby, women need the right building blocks. Apart from the extra iron needed to produce the extra haemoglobin, women need extra calcium, vitamin A and folic acid to build up their babies' bones, skin and nervous tissue. As this book is on anaemia, I'll concentrate on the iron, but it is vital for you, if you are pregnant, to ensure that you are eating foods that are rich in all these 'blocks'. Just taking them as vitamin and mineral supplements without careful attention to what you are eating is not enough.

As for iron, its transfer from mother to foetus is often on a knife-edge. Throughout a pregnancy, a woman must transfer a total of 1 gram of iron to her baby for him or her to develop normally and be born without anaemia. Remember that an adult can normally only absorb 1 mg of iron a day from her food. A pregnancy lasts 280 days, which translates into 280 mg of iron – only a quarter of the needs of the developing baby, without even starting to think of Mum's needs for it. So during pregnancy your ability to absorb iron from your gut has to rise more than fourfold if you are to avoid becoming profoundly anaemic – even if you started with a high haemoglobin level.

Clearly something has to change. Pregnant women do absorb much more iron from the same food than they did before their pregnancy. Their plasma (remember that there is much more plasma in a pregnant woman's blood than before she became pregnant) contains a substance called transferrin, which binds with the iron. Lining the circulation in the placenta are special cells that 'strip' the iron from the transferrin and deliver it to the baby's circulation. The baby's bone marrow then picks it up and makes red blood cells with it.

Sounds complex? True, but it is a perfect mechanism for the mother to deliver all the iron the baby needs to build up its own stock of blood. It ensures that the baby gets around a third of the iron its mother has absorbed from her food. However, the consequence of this is that, while the baby is sucking up so much iron from the placenta, if the mother isn't consuming enough foods that are rich in iron she will rapidly become truly anaemic. Her baby will not only take up most of the iron she consumes in her food, but will also drain the iron stores in her liver. Over the pregnancy she will lose just under one-tenth of her liver stores of iron. Most women who have high iron stores before conception can cope with this loss, but for some, who start off with poor stores (i.e. they are bordering on anaemia), a true anaemia will follow. Their haemoglobin level will drop below 10 grams per decilitre.

If you are pregnant, how can you maximize your iron absorption from your food? What matters most is that you eat food in which the iron content is readily taken up by your circulation – food with high iron bioavailability. The food with the highest bioavailability for its iron content is red meat – but not liver – because its iron is bound inside haem molecules, and our intestine absorbs haem very easily and in high amounts, much higher than the 1 mg of iron that is the daily norm. We can take in far less iron from plant sources such as vegetables (even the spinach favoured by Popeye, so well promoted as an iron provider) than from meat. If you are a strict vegetarian, then you have one of three choices: you switch to meat-eating during the pregnancy, or you greatly step up your green vegetable intake, or you swallow iron pills.

Babies who are born of anaemic women are rarely anaemic themselves, as they have enjoyed an almost unlimited supply of iron through the placenta, but once they are living on their own they can quickly become anaemic. That is because a baby's only source of iron is its mother's milk, and if she is anaemic the milk's iron content is very low – too low to sustain the infant's bone marrow and blood-forming cells.

So there is an argument for giving pregnant women extra iron by mouth, even though they are not strictly anaemic on the usual blood tests. Taking a small amount of iron each day will help its absorption and will not cause harm. It may even help those women who are on the borderline of anaemia but whose test results don't identify their risk.

Here is the current view (from the United States, although British views are similar) on whether or not we doctors should prescribe iron during pregnancy:

> Giving iron supplements during pregnancy reduces the imbalance between the foetal needs and availability of iron from the mother's food. Even then only a fraction of the iron taken in supplements is absorbed daily, meaning that some of the mother's iron stores will be used up. Continuing iron supplements after the birth lessens the impact on the mother's iron stores, and it is reasonable to continue with them for up to eight weeks. This is particularly important for women who have had previous pregnancies, whose depleted iron stores do not recover completely between pregnancies.
>
> (Taylor et al. 1982, quoted in Bridges and Pearson 2008, p. 50)

What happens to women who go through their entire pregnancy without taking extra iron? According to studies done in Germany at the beginning of this century, in the Global

North between 8 and 14 per cent of such women are clinically iron-deficient by their delivery date, and therefore likely to have babies who may become anaemic after birth (Bergmann et al. 2002). More surprising, half of all women who don't take iron supplements during their pregnancies are diagnosed as having 'latent iron deficiency'. This is a condition, not yet classifiable as anaemia, in which the values for the substances that carry iron in the blood (transferrin and ferritin) are lower than normal. Giving iron in pill form prevents overt iron deficiency but doesn't eliminate the latent form of it.

In view of these facts, what should we do? Give every woman iron tablets, so as to prevent the fairly substantial minority from becoming anaemic, iron-deficient or even latently iron-deficient? This would mean a lot of women being given iron unnecessarily so that a few benefited. Should we try to identify the women at real risk and reassure the others that they don't need extra iron? In the meantime, should we promote meat-eating for all pregnant women? I'm only half joking about the last suggestion. Imagine the stir it would create among vegetarians and all the healthy-eating lobbies who wish us to eat less meat.

Trying to identify iron deficiency among all our pregnant women would mean the extra expense of subjecting them to specialist blood tests involving measuring transferrin and ferritin, and an even more obscure test assessing levels of what are called soluble transferrin receptors. When we consider that pregnancy is a normal part of human life and not an illness, they could never be justified.

We could go back to our old favourite, the blood slide, and actually look at the red blood cells under the microscope. When we are iron-deficient the bone marrow steps up its production of new red cells, so it pushes reticulocytes into the circulation (see Chapter 1). The reticulocyte count rises steeply, but the cells look much paler than normal red cells because they contain a much lower concentration of haemoglobin. Blood-film screening for high counts of pale reticulocytes may well be the way forward. Those with positive screening results could be chosen for extra iron treatment.

While the debate continues about iron deficiency in pregnancy and what should be done about it, we family doctors have to make practical decisions on what to offer our patients. Many of us have decided that offering all our pregnant patients a small iron supplement is common sense. How much difference it really makes to someone who is not anaemic is doubtful, but if it prevents her from sliding into an iron-deficient or latent iron-deficient state, that is a good result. And it should not harm women who really don't need it.

As for women who do become anaemic during pregnancy, what do they need? If their haemoglobin has fallen below 11 grams per decilitre, then to start with they need iron supplements. The standard first choice of drug in the United Kingdom is ferrous sulphate. As we have seen, it has a reputation for causing stomach cramps, bloating and constipation, but these problems are lessened if it is taken on an empty stomach at least half an hour separated from meals. Nevertheless, if you find that you really can't tolerate it, ferrous gluconate or ferrous fumarate are good alternatives.

Women who have very low haemoglobins, and whose anaemia is making them ill, can be offered injections of iron, but only after it has been decided that taking iron by mouth would be too slow to correct the severity of the anaemia and the woman's very low iron stores. That is usually a matter for a consultant to decide. General practitioners are wary of iron injections because of their admittedly low (less than 1 per cent), but still real, risk of causing anaphylactic shock. Iron dextran is the common injectable choice in Britain: apart from the shock risk, around one in five people who are given it have joint and muscle pains, so it is not used lightly. Usually one injection is enough: this replenishes the iron stores, and then the treatment can continue with tablets.

Folic acid (folate)-deficiency anaemia in pregnancy

One type of anaemia that arises in pregnancy, and is so common that it is sensible for all pregnant women to take a supplement to help avoid it, is folic acid (or folate) deficiency. Folic acid is classified as one of the B group of vitamins. This is not the place to explain its detailed chemistry: it is enough to know that it is essential to the formation of new red blood cells. If we are severely deficient in folic acid, the red cells we produce are faulty, in that they are much larger than normal red cells but contain less haemoglobin. However, it is rare for such a severe deficiency to occur for the first time in pregnancy: we give folic acid to pregnant women as a routine mainly to prevent the milder form of folic acid-deficiency anaemia.

Because women have to increase their own red cell production by 30 per cent, and need even more folic acid to give their developing babies enough of it to ensure that their red cells, too, are normal, pregnancy forces them to raise their everyday folic acid intake by at least 50 per cent. That's impossible for most women without taking folic acid tablets as a supplement. The calculation for how much folic acid you need, like that for iron, is straightforward. The average adult woman has between 5 and 10 mg of folic acid as a store in her liver. If she doesn't take a supplement, it will be completely used up within the first half of the pregnancy. This means that three-quarters of all women will lose most of their folic acid reserves during pregnancy. As with her iron reserves, the placenta ensures that her baby will take as much of the folic acid as it needs, so that at birth few babies are folic acid-deficient. However, if she hasn't taken folic acid during her pregnancy, by the time the baby is born Mum is severely depleted – and that could make a difference to the quality of her breast milk.

Animal studies suggest that folic acid deficiency like this at the end of pregnancy is related to toxaemia (a combination of high blood pressure and kidney failure), premature birth, low-weight babies and even stillbirth. However, we don't really know the extent of these effects in human pregnancy. The consensus is that it is best not to take the risk of raising the chances of these complications, which is another reason for the universal prescription of the vitamin in pregnancy.

Folic acid and spinal and brain development

Although these last studies were in animals, the best evidence for women to take folic acid throughout their childbearing years comes from large studies in which women wishing to conceive were given either folic acid or placebo. The trials were started because of suspicions that women who had low folic acid levels might be at higher risk than others of having babies whose spines and brains did not develop normally. This leads to spina bifida (in which the nerves in the baby's lower spine are not protected by the vertebral 'shell', leading to paralysis and incontinence) and even to anencephaly (a condition incompatible with life, in which most of the brain and the top and back of the skull are absent).

The suspicions were proven to be correct. The babies of the women who were taking folic acid at the time of conception had much lower rates of spinal and brain defects at birth than the babies of mothers given placebo (Czeizel and Dudas 1992; MRC Vitamin Study Research Group 1991; Eskes 1997). The problem with these studies is that women don't usually suspect that they may be pregnant until about three or four weeks after the date of conception. By this time the spine, brain and skull are already forming, and if the mother lacks folic acid the damage is done. Starting folic acid four weeks after conception is too late to avoid potential harm for the babies of women whose levels of the vitamin are already low. That's why, for many years now, women wishing to have children have been advised in Britain to take a small dose of folic acid every day to minimize the risk of spinal and brain problems for their babies.

Folic acid-deficiency anaemia can occur quite separately from pregnancy. It is related to another vitamin-deficiency anaemia, pernicious anaemia, and can occasionally be confused with it. I deal with these two anaemias in Chapter 5.

5

Folic acid-deficiency anaemia and pernicious anaemia

Folic acid-deficiency anaemia

Sam's case

At 22, Sam decided to take a year off after graduating from university. It seemed a good idea to broaden his horizons and see the world before settling into a job in industry in Britain. He backpacked through Laos, Cambodia, Vietnam and Thailand before coming home early because of 'the runs'. Most of his fellow backpackers had had diarrhoea at some time during their travels and, although feeling quite ill, Sam thought that once he arrived back home it would quickly settle.

It didn't. He had days when he had stomach pains that almost overwhelmed him, and others when they weren't so bad. But the diarrhoea continued, he began to lose his appetite (a very unusual experience for him) and he lost more than two stones in weight. His motions, which he passed twice or three times a day, were bulky, frothy and offensive. He wasn't one for going to his doctor, but at last he had to give in.

At that first surgery visit Sam looked pale and thin. His abdomen was tender, but this was one of his good days, and there was nothing abnormal to feel in it. His doctor asked him for a sample of his stools, as he suspected a typhoid-like infection, and took a spot haemoglobin test. The reading was only 7 grams per decilitre. He admitted Sam to the regional tropical infection ward (every region in the UK now has one) and awaited the outcome of further tests.

The microbiologists couldn't find an infectious bacterium

or virus in the stools, but Sam continued to pass loose motions three times a day. His haemoglobin was confirmed at 7, and his red cells were much larger and paler than normal. The diagnosis of tropical sprue was made, and he was faced with a long recovery period that lasted many months. He was unable to work for almost a year.

Tropical sprue is thought to be caused by an as yet un-identified virus. It is widespread in the Caribbean, in India and in Southeast Asia, where Sam had picked it up, probably from a fellow backpacker. He admitted that conditions were not always hygienic, and that diarrhoea was almost accepted wherever he had travelled.

In sprue the whole of the small intestine is inflamed and unable to digest fats and carbohydrates, which, combined with the huge loss of fluid each day, quickly leads to severe malnutrition. It is also unable to absorb folic acid, so that a folic acid-deficiency anaemia is virtually inevitable. Sam needed to eat high-calorie foods despite his lack of appe-tite, and at the same time take a daily folic acid supplement. Under the care of an expert dietician and with the benefit of the folic acid, he slowly improved. The sprue eventually died down, he put on weight, and his haemoglobin was up to 11 grams per decilitre within two months.

Folic acid-deficiency anaemia can accompany any illness that interferes with digestion from the small intestine. It is common in coeliac disease, alongside the iron deficiency described in Eileen's case in Chapter 3. We see it most often in alcohol overuse, in which poor eating habits combined with liver disease lead to very low folic acid levels in the blood. However, folic acid deficiency anaemia is just one of many problems initiated by alcohol abuse, and simply giving folic acid is only a small aspect of the total manage-ment of alcoholism. It must be managed with great care and tact.

Folate-deficiency anaemia can complicate treatment with prescription drugs. People with epilepsy are particularly vulnerable, as some of the drugs they take to control their seizures (anticonvulsants) can lower the ability of the bowel to digest folic acid. Among these are phenobarbitone (phenobarbital), phenytoin and primidone. The anaemia takes years to develop but, just as with Sam's case, the red cells look large and distorted under the microscope. The long time between starting the drugs and the onset of the anaemia can make it difficult to connect the two, but everyone taking an anticonvulsant should be aware that they may develop anaemia. The answer for them is not just to take iron (their iron stores are normal) but to take a daily dose of folic acid. This rapidly reverses the anaemia and makes them feel better very quickly.

Some anticancer drugs also produce folic acid-deficiency anaemia, but the cancer team are usually very well aware of the possibility and will identify the early changes before they become serious. Rather than stopping the drug, the correct course is to give extra folic acid. The same goes for methotrexate, a drug that has had great success in treating rheumatoid arthritis, severe psoriasis and exfoliative dermatitis (in which there is excessive skin inflammation and loss). Again, the answer is to continue the treatment, but to add folic acid to it.

Folic acid tablets are remarkably free of side effects: the usual maximum dose is 5 mg a day, but over-the-counter tablet strengths of up to 0.6 mg are usually more than enough to reverse anaemia, unless it is particularly severe or your ability to absorb it is extremely restricted by bowel disease. In the latter (extremely rare) case, injections of 5 mg per millilitre are given.

Pernicious anaemia

In his day, George Bernard Shaw was as much a public figure as the most famous film and stage and television stars of today. He was known, even hero-worshipped, for his wit and his plays, many of which are still relevant and topical 100 years after his heyday. *The Doctor's Dilemma* and *Mrs Warren's Profession* could have been written today. He was also known for his rampant vegetarianism: he never hid his distaste for eating animals and for those who did eat them. Yet like many modern celebrities, he had a guilty secret. On each day of the last 50 years of his long life (he lived into his 90s) he ate a large meal of raw liver. George had pernicious anaemia, and raw liver was the only way it could be treated in the first half of the twentieth century. Naturally he and his entourage kept this quiet from the press, who would have had a field day with his animal-eating habits had they known.

People with pernicious anaemia today don't have to face raw liver. An injection once a month is enough to keep them completely healthy, and it is acceptable to the most rigorous vegetarians.

Sean's case

I met Sean for the first time when he was in his late 20s. Our practice was based on a fishing village on the southwest coast of Scotland. Sean could trace his fishing ancestry back three centuries, and was at his happiest when living by, or working on, the sea. That first meeting wasn't a medical one. He and his uncle had invited me to join them for 'a day at the herring'. Partly it was to show me how hard they worked, and partly, I suspect, they wanted to see their doctor sick for a change: they wanted to get their own back. It was the hardest physical work I have ever done – even harder than the day I spent down a mine. I never moan about the price of fish or coal.

The point of this story? On that day, Sean was a picture of strength and health. He could haul the heaviest of nets on board, and without a qualm could leap easily and nimbly from one boat to another (a necessity in the job of ring-netting herring). Sure-footed as a mountain goat and as strong as an ox, he should certainly have strolled into the future without a care.

I didn't see Sean medically for five years after that day. When he came into the surgery, I was shocked. He was pale and stooped. He felt tired all the time, was breathless on the slightest exertion, often felt his heart beating hard and fast in his chest and, when he went to bed at night, could hear whistling in his ears that prevented him from sleeping. He hadn't been to sea for several months. His ankles had started swelling and he was now worried that he had a heart problem. What worried him most, however, was that his mother thought he 'was going the way his father had'. His symptoms, his mother said, were similar to his dad's, and his dad had died suddenly in his late 30s.

Talking to Sean, I was struck that he was hesitating as he talked. He was not his usual calm self. At one point he became irritated by my questions, then he apologized for his rudeness and started to cry. He apologized for that too, as he dried his eyes. Of course, I reassured him and put him at his ease. I asked him if he could think of any other problems that might be relevant.

'Yes,' he said, 'I'm getting pins and needles in my feet, and my toes seem to be numb. And if I try to file my nails with an emery board, it feels really odd – it's a horrible sensation.'

I didn't need to ask him more questions. A brief examination told me the rest of his story. He had a large, smooth, shiny tongue, but it wasn't sore as it might have been with iron or folic acid deficiency. He was very pale, in spite of his outdoor life as a fisherman. His pulse was fast and bounding.

His ankles were a little swollen: when I pressed my thumb into the skin it left a dimple that was slow to fill up.

The most telling signs were in his feet. When he shut his eyes and let me move his great toe up and down, he didn't know in which direction it was bent. He couldn't feel a tuning fork vibrating on the bones of his feet. Scratching the soles of his feet made his big toes arch upwards instead of curling down, as they should have. A pinprick blood sample showed a haemoglobin of 4.7 grams per decilitre. He had less than a third of the oxygen-carrying capacity that he should have had. The history was so clear and the examination result so precise that I felt I could make the diagnosis on the spot, but I took two further blood samples for the laboratory staff to make sure. The first was for a microscopic examination of a blood smear, and the second for a blood vitamin B12 level.

The smear confirmed that he had far fewer red cells than normal. At an average of 105 cubic micrometres in volume, they were much larger than red cells in normal conditions and were very pale, with far less haemoglobin in them than normal. Most of them were oval rather than the normal round shape. His vitamin B12 level was well below the lower limit of normal for our hospital laboratory. There was no doubt that he had pernicious anaemia.

On learning that the diagnosis had been proven I was hugely relieved, because today pernicious anaemia is very easily treated. After a single injection of the missing vitamin (vitamin B12 is also called cyanocobalamin or simply cobalamin), Sean felt miraculously better. He has since had an injection once a month, his haemoglobin is now 14.5 grams per decilitre, and he can expect to live a normal and long life. He is back at sea, though the herring have gone, perhaps for ever, from the Clyde estuary, and he is now a lobsterman.

What we know about pernicious anaemia

Why did such a healthy man develop pernicious anaemia in his early 30s? One clue lay in his father's early death. Although we had no notes from his father's time, how he died strongly suggested that he, too, had pernicious anaemia. The tendency towards it is inherited. Looking further back in his family history, Sean unearthed stories of great-uncles who had similar illnesses.

This was strong evidence that Sean's case was inherited and that he had an autoimmune disease: as he entered adult life his immune system, for some yet unknown reason, began to misidentify as 'foreign' the cells (they are called parietal cells) that organize the uptake of vitamin B12 in the stomach. Once misidentified like this, these cells were destroyed, just as the immune system would destroy an invading bacterium or virus. It is a process that takes years to complete, but once these specialized stomach-lining cells were all gone Sean was left without any way of taking up vitamin B12 normally from his food.

Vitamin B12 is unique among all our vitamins in that it doesn't get absorbed in the state in which it exists in our food. The parietal cells which produce the acid that starts off the process of digestion also produce a substance called intrinsic factor. It combines with vitamin B12 to produce a complex chemical called transcobalamin II (TC II), which can pass through the gut wall into the circulation. Without intrinsic factor there can be no TC II, and the vitamin (cobalamin – hence transcobalamin) can't be transported to the bone marrow to play its part in producing new red blood cells. The cells that are formed without it are exactly those described in Sean's blood smear – large, oval, very much deficient in haemoglobin, and far fewer than are needed to maintain oxygen delivery to the tissues and organs.

Cobalamin isn't just used to produce red blood cells. It is important for maintaining and renewing nerve and brain cells. Lack of it leads to a general feeling of dis-ease, emotional upsets, difficulty in concentration, and those abnormalities in the long nerves to the limbs that produced the pins and needles, numbness and odd reflex reactions that were so evident in Sean's case.

The whistling in the ears was a pointer to his severe anaemia. The carotid arteries on each side of the neck carry more than two-thirds of the blood supply from the heart to the head (the rest comes from the basilar artery in front of the spine). On their journey they pass very close to the middle ear. When anaemia becomes as severe as Sean's, his circulation has to pump what remains of his haemoglobin much faster and at higher pressure through the carotids. The sound of the rushing blood is amplified in the middle-ear chamber – my old ENT tutor likened it to the effect in the whispering gallery in St Paul's Cathedral – and it is picked up by the inner ear as a whistle. It is less noticeable in the daytime, but is much more obvious at night when trying to sleep.

This type of 'whistle' or 'roar' – the noise can appear as either – is one of the symptoms a doctor will pick up on as a pointer to severe anaemia. When it starts later in life many people just put it down to ageing, and ignore it. Or they have heard about tinnitus and think it's something for which nothing can be done. Both decisions can be so wrong and can delay the true diagnosis. So if you have noises in your ears when you are trying to sleep, and you notice them from time to time during quiet periods during the daytime, please let your doctor know about it. Never assume that it is an inevitable or untreatable part of ageing.

Sean's inherited autoimmune form of pernicious anaemia has a few extra drawbacks. As the stomach loses its intrinsic factor-producing parietal cells, it loses its acid production too.

For a reason that's still difficult to understand, the change in the cells predisposes them to turning cancerous, so that if you have Sean's type of pernicious anaemia you will probably be asked to attend a regular follow-up clinic to identify any subtle changes in the stomach lining well before they turn into malignancy. So far, Sean is clear of such complications, but from what we know now about his father's last illness, this may have been his cause of death. The family are aware of this, and Sean's two sons will be checked when they reach their 20s.

Another aspect of autoimmune pernicious anaemia is that it is sometimes linked to other autoimmune disorders. In particular, the thyroid gland may be affected, which at first stimulates the thyroid into over- and then to under-activity. So Sean's blood is also checked for the beginning of antibodies (a sign of autoimmune activity) against his thyroid gland. There is also a higher than usual risk of changes in skin colour in a condition called vitiligo, where antibodies form that are specifically against the melanin-producing pigment cells in the skin. This leaves patches of white skin that stand out against the surrounding skin, regardless of the usual skin colour. So far, Sean has been free of these complications, and we hope he remains so.

How did George Bernard Shaw manage without injections? Raw liver does contain large amounts of vitamin B12, and if you eat a lot of it a very small proportion of it is absorbed, an even smaller amount of which the body can use to make red cells. It must have been purgatory for him, and he probably was relatively anaemic despite it, which possibly accounted for his famous irascibility and languor. He was also lucky not to suffer from vitamin A overdose. Animal liver contains high levels of vitamin A, overdose of which can cause severe skin problems, and GBS must have been at high risk of them. When vitamin B12 was at last found to be the cause, liver treatment for pernicious anaemia was abandoned overnight.

Sean's type of pernicious anaemia was inherited, but there is a form of irritation of the stomach lining caused by infection (with the ulcer-causing bacterium *Helicobacter pylori*) that we acquire, mainly when we are children, that can lead years later to low vitamin B12 levels. Called chronic atrophic gastritis, it slowly replaces the parietal cells by a sheet of inflammation, causing the acid levels in the stomach to fall. We need the acid to release vitamin B12 from our food, so that without it there is not enough free vitamin to combine with the intrinsic factor that the stomach is still producing. If you have chronic atrophic gastritis, you slowly lose your stores of vitamin B12. This form of vitamin B12 deficiency is less obvious and less severe than the true pernicious anaemia seen in Sean, but it can still make people feel severely under par.

Happily we can cure *Helicobacter* infections, and greatly improve chronic atrophic gastritis, by prescribing a month's course of combined antibiotics and acid-reducing drugs. Although it is not officially recommended, some doctors have found that adding injections of vitamin B12 to the treatment of patients recovering from atrophic gastritis makes them feel much better sooner than with the anti-*Helicobacter* drugs alone. I can't recommend it in a book like this, but I know several colleagues who have found the boost that vitamin B12 injections give so important to their patients that they use it almost as a pick-me-up in other conditions too. I feel that is going too far.

Given that loss of the area of stomach that produces acid and intrinsic factor almost eliminates our uptake of vitamin B12 from food, older people who have had parts of their stomach removed because of ulcer disease (I mentioned earlier that this stopped in the 1980s) are at risk of becoming anaemic over the next two or three decades. Because of this, when we see people in their 60s and older with severe anaemia, we make sure that they haven't had stomach surgery in their early adult life as this can lead to anaemia almost identical to classical pernicious anaemia, much like Sean's.

Which brings me appropriately, in the next chapter, to the subject of anaemia in older people.

6

Anaemia in older people

Growing older is never straightforward. We tend to collect illnesses, so that few of us reach our late 60s without having to take regular medicines for something. Among the afflictions of older age is anaemia, but it is debatable whether there is a true 'anaemia of old age' that arises simply because we are older, independently of any other complicating condition. Routine blood testing in older people, say from 60 onwards, shows that more of them are anaemic than are their younger counterparts. But for how many of them is the anaemia simply an inevitable part of their ageing, and for how many is it a symptom of an unrelated illness? It is vital to know, because, as with younger adults, if there is a cause that can be corrected, we have to find it. There is no upper age barrier beyond which we don't need to investigate the cause of a case of anaemia.

So let us deal with the 'ageing thing', and get it out of the way. Does old age in itself predispose to anaemia? Does our bone marrow gradually become less efficient at producing red cells filled with the correct concentration of haemoglobin? If it does, then if we find that someone aged 80 is anaemic, we will assume that this is normal, that we don't need to find the cause, and we can simply decide to treat it with iron tablets and advise on eating well.

We are well used to other organs 'wearing out' with age. Arthritis, for example, is looked upon as the result of wearing out of cartilage in the knees and hips, due to years of having to bear the weight of the body. As we age we can't repair the joint surfaces as well as when we were younger. Does the bone marrow act in the same way? It replaces old red cells with new ones: if age causes that system to slow down or be less efficient, anaemia is bound to follow.

However, there is no evidence that this happens. A group of healthy 88-year-olds volunteered to have their haemoglobins measured and have bone marrow samples examined (Nilsson-Ehle et al. 1995). Most of them had normal haemoglobin levels, with only a few verging on the edge of mild anaemia. Admittedly, there were slightly fewer red cell precursor cells (the cells that form the red cells) but there were no consistent abnormalities in them that would suggest damage related to ageing. The authors concluded that there were bone marrow changes in 88-year-olds that meant that they were producing fewer red cells, but that they did not amount to such severe loss of cells as would lead to anaemia. Anaemia, they wrote, is not the norm even in the 'older elderly'.

This conclusion is supported by another study of over 1,000 people in whom the average haemoglobin levels remained high up to the age of at least 85 (Timiras and Brownstein 1987), and by another showing that healthy people living at home with good eating habits maintain their normal haemoglobin levels (Olivares et al. 2000).

The phrase 'good eating habits' is crucial, because rates of anaemia do rise in the elderly, and by far the commonest cause is poor nutrition, particularly among people living at home alone. Not far behind poor eating habits as a cause of anaemia are chronic kidney disease and chronic inflammation caused by arthritis, iron deficiency due to internal bleeding, and vitamin B12 and folic acid deficiency.

I have dealt with iron deficiency in Chapter 3, but it is worth repeating that if we find someone in his or her 70s or 80s with iron-deficiency anaemia we should never assume that it has been caused by a poor diet. Even in very old age, bleeding from bowel cancer and stomach ulcers is top of the list of causes, and their chances of cure in older age are as high as in younger people. Regardless of someone's age we must investigate all cases of anaemia. Anti-*Helicobacter* treatment of stomach and duodenal ulcers, for example, is as successful in eradicating the germ and stopping the bleeding in the very old as it is in the young.

One aspect of anaemia in older people that does differentiate them from the young is that their condition affects them much more severely. They become much more tired and are much less able to perform their usual household tasks than a younger person with the same level of anaemia. Their lack of energy causes them to feel much more 'down', and it can be the sole cause of their lack of enjoyment of the life to which they had so much looked forward before retiring.

When we develop anaemia in older age we become weaker and unsteadier, so that we fall more easily than before. Sometimes it is a fall that leads to the diagnosis of anaemia, and if you are anaemic when you fall, and perhaps break a thigh, the road to recovery and healing is much longer and rockier than it would otherwise have been. Anaemia is one of the complications of fractures in the old that puts them at a higher risk of dying from them.

So how do we treat older people we find to be anaemic? The first principle is to look upon it in exactly the same way as we would with younger patients who have the same diagnosis. We need to find the cause. The American authors of one of the medical textbooks on anaemia state that no specific 'anaemia of old age' exists. From a practical point of view, doctors have to agree with that.

Step number 1 for a family doctor like me is to go into how well people are eating and looking after themselves. Widowers are notorious for eating poorly: it is common for them not to bother to cook and to subsist on sandwiches, fast-food meals and tea. Meat, vegetables and fruit make rare appearances on their table, if they ever bother to sit at one. Iron deficiency, folic acid deficiency and even vitamin B12 deficiency follow this pattern of eating (really, of not eating) almost as surely as night follows day. The answer to their problem is to organize healthy eating for them. In the United Kingdom we have systems, publicly and privately funded, to cater for them. Often it is simply a matter of making sure they get one good meal a day. Once the better eating habits have been established the anaemia will reverse, and they feel better before we even note that the haemoglobin has risen. Helping people eat more healthily at home or with others in day-care units brings them out of themselves, so their mental health improves alongside their physical well-being.

However, simply finding that older people haven't been eating well enough isn't an excuse for not investigating further. A few extra blood tests may point to other reasons for the low haemoglobin level that will not respond positively to better general care alone. One of these is chronic kidney disease. Edward's story is typical.

Anaemia of kidney disease: Edward's case

Edward Simpson was 63 when he moved home to the countryside on retiring from a mainly sedentary job in a busy city office. He had not felt the need, nor had he had the time, to visit his city doctor while he was working. His new home was on the outskirts of our seaside village, and he was looking forward to enjoying a garden (he had lived in a flat) and a spot of sea fishing, something that he had done in his youth and wanted to take up again.

Naturally, he had to transfer his medical records to our health centre, and he was a little surprised that it involved more than just dropping in his medical cards. Our nurse gave him an appointment for a well-man check, two weeks ahead.

By that time, with the garden cleared of weeds and the boat ready for the sea, Edward was feeling quite tired. The extra physical effort put into them had made him recognize that he wasn't as fit as he had thought he was. So when the nurse asked him how he felt generally, he admitted to needing to become a bit fitter but said that he had always been healthy. His only previous problem had been a urinary infection 15 years before – that had been the last time he had consulted a doctor.

For someone in his 60s this was unusual. By the time they reach Edward's age many men are seeing their doctors once or twice every two years or so. Some are taking regular prescription medicines for chronic conditions such as high blood pressure or arthritis: others are simply being seen to make sure that they are continuing to be well, so that they are on the annual list for bowel and prostate checks, or for flu injections.

So our nurse might have been forgiven for assuming that it was natural that when someone of 60-plus switched from a seated to an active lifestyle he would find the change a challenge to his fitness levels. She didn't make that mistake.

All new patients to doctors' lists are put through thorough medical checks, and these include blood tests. Edward's finger-prick test showed a haemoglobin of only 10 grams per decilitre. This was as much a surprise to the nurse as to him. She ordered a raft of extra tests to try to find the reason, and passed him on to the duty doctor.

Among the tests were those to check for prostate health (PSA), for any sign of chronic inflammation (CRP) and for kidney disease (eGFR). A rise in PSA levels (the letters stand for prostate specific antigen) in men may indicate prostate cancer or infections. CRP stands for C-reactive protein, rises in which indicate chronic inflammatory disease such as rheumatoid arthritis or a chronic infection somewhere in the body. eGFR stands for estimated glomerular filtration rate: it is a measure of how well the kidneys are managing to deal with the production and excretion of urine.

Edward's PSA and CRP were normal, so we could rule out prostate and chronic inflammation as the direct cause of anaemia, but his eGFR was surprisingly low. The eGFR is calculated from a complex formula that takes into account the blood level of a substance called creatinine, your age and sex. How to calculate it is beyond the scope of this book: it is enough here to state that a normal eGFR is 90 or more millilitres per minute per 1.3 square metres of body surface. An eGFR of 60 to 89 represents mild – or stage 2 – chronic kidney disease. From 30 to 59 the person has stage 3, or moderate disease; below that the disease is classified as severe.

Edward's eGFR was 51, well into stage 3 chronic renal failure, yet he had had no symptoms of kidney disease. He never had to get up at night to pass urine, he had no swelling of the ankles, he had not noticed that he had had to pass urine more often during the day, or that he was passing either more or less urine than before. In other words, his kidney disease had come out of the blue for him and for his medical team. The probable cause was chronic glomerulonephritis, an inflammation of the kidney cells that had started in his late teens or early adult life and that had continued to worsen imperceptibly over many years. That 'urinary infection' of 15 years previously might have been a clue to it.

His story is by no means unusual. Since we started to use the eGFR test to check on kidney function in healthy adults in Britain, we have found that around 4 to 10 per cent of all those tested over 55 years of age will fall into the 'moderate' group. That is, they have eGFR levels under 60: put another way, they have lost 40 per cent of their kidney function.

This sounds very serious, and it is, but not in the way that you might think. Naturally, whenever we have to tell people that they have moderate chronic kidney disease, everyone asks the obvious next question: 'Will I have to have dialysis or a kidney transplant?' Fewer than 2 per cent of them eventually reach the stage, with an eGFR below 15, at which first dialysis and then transplant is needed. Most people stay in the 'moderate' stage for the rest of their lives: they avoid the more serious phase of kidney failure, but they have other health risks that they must be helped to avoid, or at least postpone. Among them is heart disease.

The connection between chronic kidney disease (CKD) and heart disease is striking: men and women with moderate CKD are at much higher risk of heart attacks and strokes than are people with normal kidneys, and the more severe their CKD, the higher their risk. When the kidneys begin to lose their ability to filter away waste products and to produce urine, automatic mechanisms switch on to try to push more blood through them. The aim, of course, is to improve the flow of blood through the delicate organs, the glomeruli, that concentrate and filter away the waste materials from the blood while retaining everything we need. It is obviously an extremely complex system, and the higher blood pressure tends to damage it.

That is unfortunate, because the damage leads eventually to even poorer kidney function, and therefore to the message to increase the pressure further. A vicious circle continues, producing the slow deterioration seen in so many CKD patients over decades. The high blood pressure leads directly to an overgrowth (the medical term is hypertrophy) of the heart muscles, so that the heart becomes enlarged. Eventually the heart can become so large that the coronary arteries that supply it with oxygen can no longer cope. The hypertrophic muscle is then unable to contract efficiently and cannot continue to maintain the necessary pumping action. This state is called heart failure: and in the past it was the usual cause of death in chronic kidney disease.

Now add anaemia to the CKD story. If you are anaemic your heart needs to beat even faster, and with more force, to maintain your body's (and your heart's) oxygen needs. If your heart is already overgrowing, anaemia will add to that stress: it may even be the initial cause of the hypertrophy. And the two disorders, CKD and anaemia, are directly connected. It is no coincidence that most CKD patients are also anaemic – and if the anaemia is correctly treated, they can reduce their heart risks almost down to the normal level for people of the same age with no kidney problem.

Happily, today we are well aware of all the risks from CKD and its accompanying anaemia. We have an array of excellent drugs to lower blood pressure, use of which has been proved not only to improve kidney function, by maintaining good circulation through it, but also to reduce the heart complications.

EPO (Erythropoietin)

Treating the anaemia, however, is not just a matter of giving CKD patients iron. To understand why, we have to know about erythropoietin, or EPO. You will have heard of it, but not in the context of anaemia. EPO became notorious in the 1990s as a means by which athletes could build up their oxygen-carrying capacity. Injections of EPO stimulate the bone marrow to increase its production of new red blood cells, so that an athlete who had a previous haemoglobin of 15 grams per decilitre and a red cell count of 5 million per microlitre could use it to boost them to 18 and 6 respectively. This would give a huge advantage in stamina and in energy use, especially for long-distance running and in other endurance sports, and is obviously cheating.

EPO is a natural hormone. Healthy kidneys produce it as a response to any fall in red cell and haemoglobin levels: our bone marrow picks up the rising EPO levels in our blood and responds by making more red cells, passing them on into the bloodstream. It is a constant feedback system: when the kidneys detect that there are enough red cells in the circulation, they reduce their EPO output and the marrow slows down its production. The marrow depends on the kidneys for its ability to maintain blood levels, and if the kidneys were to stop producing EPO, anaemia would result.

That is exactly what has happened in the anaemia of chronic kidney disease. Quite early in the disease, the kidneys begin to lose their ability to produce EPO. The bone marrow slows its production of cells, and the anaemia follows.

It is obvious from this that it would be of little use simply to give people like Edward iron tablets, or even extra vitamins such as folic acid and vitamin B12, which are all involved in making red cells. If the main stimulus for the marrow to produce them has gone, the only way to correct the problem is to replace it. Luckily that is now very easy. We have the drugs that cheating athletes use, except that we prescribe them professionally, under close supervision. Medically they are called erythropoiesis-stimulating agents, or ESAs. They are available legally only on prescription, and are given by doctors or specialist nurses in injections placed just under the skin. The dose depends on how anaemic you are.

Giving an ESA to an athlete who by definition already has enough red blood cells (otherwise he or she couldn't compete) has its dangers. Increasing red cell numbers beyond the normal heightens the risk of high blood pressure as the thickening blood becomes more viscous and more difficult to pump around the body. It also makes clot formation in the smaller arteries more likely, leading directly to heart attacks and strokes, so the athletes who use it, and their coaches who condone it, are taking huge risks for their chance of fame.

But for people with CKD-related anaemia, ESAs can be a lifesaver. By pressing on the marrow's accelerator, after just one injection a host of reticulocytes (see Chapter 1) appear in the blood, showing that its effect is immediate. The anaemia quickly reverses, providing the person eats well and takes extra iron to allow the marrow to cope with the extra demand for it. How much iron is needed depends on the depth of the anaemia: your doctor will know the optimum doses of both iron and your ESA, and will review them every month to begin with, stretching them to two months later. The aim in CKD-related anaemia is to achieve a haemoglobin of 12 grams per decilitre, stop the ESA and monitor the haemoglobin from then onwards every three months. If it begins to fall again, the treatment can be restarted.

Edward responded to his ESA and iron treatment very well. Within a few days his reticulocyte count was in the teens, and he felt much better. He reached his goal of 12.5 grams per decilitre within three months. That was three years ago: his eGFR has remained steady at around 55. Best of all, his heart size has shrunk to within the normal range (it had started to increase) and his blood pressure remains normal too. He is now in little danger of a stroke or heart attack, and there seems to be no fear that his kidney disease will worsen significantly. Proper correction of his anaemia has almost certainly saved his life.

7

Anaemia in arthritis and cancer

Anaemias caused by bleeding, iron deficiency and even lack of erythropoietin are straightforward to identify and to treat. However, there are more complex causes of anaemia that we are not yet able to cure completely. Among them are the anaemias of longstanding inflammation and of cancer.

The experts classify them as the anaemias of chronic inflammation, or ACI. For many years we have known that people with inflammatory disorders such as rheumatoid arthritis, longstanding infections such as tuberculosis, and many types of cancer develop anaemia that is not simply caused by lack of iron or vitamins. They do not respond satisfactorily to iron and vitamin supplements, to healthier eating or even to the relatively low doses of erythropoietin, described in the previous chapter, that are used in chronic kidney disease. There is something about chronic debilitating illnesses that leads to anaemia despite all the usual corrections and treatments.

Since 2005, researchers have begun to be optimistic that they may be knocking at the doors of the cause. They have discovered a substance called hepcidin (Frazer et al. 2002), made in the liver, that acts on the lining cells of the duodenum to stop iron from food or pills being taken up into the bloodstream. If you have high levels of hepcidin in your liver, you simply can't digest iron, so that no matter how much of it you swallow, you won't be able to transfer it all the way to your bone marrow. Without fresh iron supplies, you will inevitably become anaemic.

Nor is it any use giving iron by injection. Normally this

would be a reasonable substitute for iron by mouth. However, high hepcidin levels in the bloodstream also block the mechanism (it is called ferroportin) for transporting iron from the blood to the bone marrow, so that the injected iron stays stubbornly in the bloodstream and can't be used by the marrow (Delaby et al. 2005).

Which leaves us with a puzzle: why should we have a mechanism that prevents us taking up iron and, even more perplexing, why does it operate in people with chronic illnesses, who need iron most? The first part of the question can be answered fairly easily. Hepcidin is just part of the system that controls uptake of iron in normal digestion. We only need a little iron every day, so hepcidin is useful for shutting down iron absorption when we have enough stores of the mineral. It is another of those feedback mechanisms upon which our bodies rely.

If that feedback mechanism goes wrong – if there is a continuous stimulus to hepcidin production that overrules the feedback loop – then hepcidin levels remain high and iron absorption stops. This is exactly what happens in chronic inflammation and cancers. Our body's immune system, in its attempt to combat the abnormal chemicals that exist in such diseases, produces substances called inflammatory cytokines. The details are beyond the scope of this book, but suffice it to say that there are at least three (they go by the names of IL-6, IL-1alpha and IL-1beta) that are now known to induce the liver to go into hepcidin overproduction mode. Only one (it is called TNF-alpha) has so far been shown to cut hepcidin production.

Unfortunately, it is not yet possible to give people with ACI a specific anti-hepcidin treatment. IL-6 is the most important of the hepcidin-inducing cytokines: high levels of it are found in a host of tumours, including breast, lung, prostate and ovarian cancers, and in lymphomas and leukaemias. If we could block its action on hepcidin, would that help to cure the anaemias that are almost inevitable in these malignancies, or would it, by blocking a possible anticancer effect, simply cause tumours to develop faster? This is just one of the quandaries facing the researchers and the doctors looking after cancer patients. TNF-alpha sounded promising at first, but it stops the bone marrow cells from responding to erythropoietin and would just substitute one form of anaemia for another.

By now you will have gathered that ACI is extremely complex and cannot be treated easily. In the past the only answer was to give blood transfusions when the anaemia became so bad that it was severely affecting the person's quality of life. Transfusion does work well, and if you are severely anaemic it is the only way in which you can feel better almost instantaneously. Up to the 1980s, before the horror stories of people being infected with HIV and hepatitis viruses almost destroyed the blood transfusion services, about 10 per cent of all blood transfusions were given to people with severe ACI, most of them with cancers.

Blood transfusion today is much safer than it was, in that there are safety mechanisms in place to prevent infection through donated blood, but it has other drawbacks. Remember that in Chapter 3 I wrote about the difficulty the body has in getting rid of iron? This is a particular problem for blood transfusions. With each successive transfusion, more iron is loaded into our livers, and into other organs, and this can lead eventually to heart and liver failure. And no blood donor sample is an exact match for the recipient's blood, so that people who have repeated transfusions develop immunity to them – the transfusion experts can no longer find donor blood that someone can still tolerate. Repeated blood transfusions for ACI anaemia are now almost abandoned, except for people who have failed to respond to all other treatments.

Erythropoietin is the partial answer. At the time cancer experts were looking for an alternative to transfusion, there was the first true success in drug genetic engineering. It was the result of manipulating the structure of the erythropoietin (EPO) mentioned earlier in the treatment of the anaemia of chronic kidney disease. The first patients with CKD who were given it responded so well that cancer experts and rheumatologists struggling to find an answer to their patients' anaemias tried it out on them. The hepcidin story suggested that it might not work (hepcidin does not feature in CKD), but three erythropoiesis-stimulating agents (ESAs) have since been given official approval because of their quite surprising success.

The trick in overcoming the hepcidin problem, apparently, is that it takes a short time for it to combine with the iron coming in from the gut. If a dose of an ESA is given immediately after a substantial oral dose of iron, some of the iron will escape the hepcidin mechanism and transfer into the bone marrow.

In cancer-associated anaemias, the ESA is given as an injection just under the skin, usually once every three weeks to coincide with the patient's regular review. The aim is to increase the haemoglobin by 1–2 grams per decilitre between injections. An improvement of this order usually means the patient feels much better within a month. Three-quarters of people who gain by 1 gram in the first month go on to do well in the long term.

Why treat cancer-related anaemias?

Questions that are often raised (usually by someone with no personal or family experience of cancer) about people who have an incurable cancer include asking why we try to treat their anaemia at all, particularly if the treatment is an added expense. Will treating their anaemia make them feel any better or prolong their life in any quality?

Severe anaemia in cancer – or, for that matter, in other chronic life-changing illnesses – leaves you extremely tired and often very breathless. Constant mind-numbing fatigue is a desperate state and is often the cause of suicide. Being unable to breathe deeply, slowly or satisfyingly is similarly cruel. If we can relieve both of these symptoms we should use all we have to hand to do so. There are plenty of studies on just this subject.

For example, in two studies involving more than 4,000 cancer patients being treated at home, improving their haemoglobin levels simply from 11 to 12 grams per decilitre made the biggest improvement in their sense of well-being. This suggests that we shouldn't wait until the anaemia becomes severe before we start to treat it. Dr P. Stone and colleagues reported that half of their patients said that fatigue was severely spoiling their enjoyment in life, yet more than half of them had never discussed it with their carers or clinic staff. They had assumed that nothing could be done about it. In another study, 90 per cent of cancer patients said that fatigue had made them alter their daily routine, such as walking, cleaning and other household chores. Of this 90 per cent, 60 per cent felt that fatigue was worse to bear than nausea, pain and depression (Stone et al. 2000).

Correcting anaemia in cancer can improve your quality of life even if the tumour is continuing to grow and the cancer spreading, a fact, as shown by several authors, which strongly supports the point that the fatigue is not the direct result of the cancer but of the anaemia itself.

So should everyone with anaemia due to cancer or to long-term chronic inflammation be given an ESA? Two points must be made. One is that 40 per cent of people don't respond to it. They may need a transfusion schedule that minimizes their risk of side effects from repeated transfusions. The other is that there is no evidence that treating the anaemia prolongs the patient's life. Some trials have reported that there is an excess of deaths from thrombosis (blood clots) in patients receiving EPOs, but the largest survey of 57 trials in 9,000 patients shows no difference in life survival between those given an ESA and those without one (Bohlius et al. 2006). It seems that if we have cancer, treating the anaemia that almost always accompanies it offers us a better quality of life and relief from the ever-present tiredness, but it will not prolong our lives. However, this is still a very big advantage over the old attitude of 'letting things be'.

8

Sickle-cell anaemia and thalassaemia

In 1910, Dr James Herrick reported on the problems of a student in his care from Grenada in the West Indies. The young man's main complaints were of longstanding tiredness and lack of energy, but he also admitted to periods when his joints hurt, and at other times he would have bouts of very severe pain that were general – all over his body. Examining him, Dr Herrick's only abnormal finding was that the whites of his patient's eyes were slightly yellow, suggesting very mild jaundice. The big surprise came when he examined a smear of the young man's blood. His red cells looked strange: they were crescent-shaped or sickle-shaped. They were also fewer than normal, so that the young man was severely anaemic.

Dr Herrick called this new disease 'sickle-cell anaemia'. We don't know how that first patient progressed under Dr Herrick's care, but the course of his illness was probably fairly stormy. We know, of course, much more now about sickle-cell disease (the name was changed from sickle-cell anaemia when it was recognized that it affected much more than simply the red cell count) than did Dr Herrick, but the problems faced by those with the condition remain the same. Prominent among them is chronic anaemia.

Writing in 2008 about sickle-cell disease in the USA, Drs Kenneth Bridges and Howard Pearson state that it 'remains one of the most challenging disorders in medicine'. It affects 80,000 Americans, so that it is the commonest cause of serious anaemia in the United States. In sub-Saharan Africa and in India it is even more common: in the United Kingdom, too, it is of serious concern to our people of African and South Asian origin.

Why should such a strange disorder have survived in such large numbers of people? The key is in their African and Asian origins. Malaria parasites cannot survive and multiply within sickle cells: they need normal red cells to complete their complex lifecycle. Over millennia, people with sickle cells had the advantage of being resistant to malaria, so they were fitter than their suffering friends with normal red cells. Darwin's law of the fittest surviving kept the 'sicklers' alive into the present age. Sadly, possession of sickle cells isn't an unmixed blessing, and in non-malarial areas it is a huge drawback, one symptom of which is a pattern of fatigue, discomfort and pain like that suffered by Dr Herrick's original patient.

We have known since 1956, from the work of Dr Vernon Ingram of the United Kingdom's Medical Research Council, that sickle cells are the result of an abnormal haemoglobin gene – for the purists it is the beta-haemoglobin molecule that is affected. Not all sickle cases show the same mutation: there are several types of abnormality, which partly explains the wide range in sickle-cell disease severity. To be pedantic, sickle-cell disease is not a single entity, but a group of similarly inherited disorders linked by the fact that their end result is the sickle-shaped red cell.

Oddly, although sickle-cell disease is inherited, it doesn't affect the newborn. That's because during our life inside the womb our bone marrow makes foetal haemoglobin rather than adult haemoglobin, and foetal haemoglobin is not affected by the genetic mutation. As the baby continues to survive on foetal haemoglobin for the first four months of life, sickling only appears after that time, after foetal haemoglobin disappears and adult haemoglobin kicks in. Parents may not suspect that something is wrong until the first episode of illness, usually after their baby is nine months old. The first signs are painful swellings in the hands and feet, conveniently called 'hand-foot syndrome'. From the second birthday onwards the children start to have bouts of pain in the limbs, back and abdomen: how severe they are and how often they happen varies greatly from child to child.

Children who start with hand-foot syndrome before they are one year old and who have a haemoglobin below 7 grams per decilitre by the age of two are faced with severe continuing illness throughout their childhood. They are the children who need to be considered for bone marrow stem cell transplant from a healthy sibling – about which more later.

Tragically, children with sickle-cell disease face high risks of severe, often life-threatening complications throughout their lives. This is not the place to go into detail about them, but they include:

- repeated strokes caused by the abnormal cells clumping and blocking arteries in the brain. One in five children with sickle-cell anaemia will show areas of brain damage on magnetic resonance imaging (MRI) scans. Only repeated blood transfusions can prevent stroke recurrence in them;
- 'aplastic crisis', in which infection with a virus causing the common childhood illness 'fifth disease' leads to shutdown of red cell production by the bone marrow;
- acute splenic sequestration, in which the spleen suddenly enlarges as it removes massive numbers of red cells from the circulation, leading to shock, anaemia in which the haemoglobin can be as low as 2 to 4 grams per decilitre, and death, if it is not treated urgently with blood transfusion and fluid replacement. The spleen is usually removed to prevent future episodes, which may leave children with difficulties in fighting infection.

This catalogue makes sickle-cell disease sound extremely serious, and it is exactly that for those children who suffer the above complications. However, some children have such mild symptoms that their sickling may not be diagnosed until they are adults. Mild disease doesn't necessarily remain mild. Puberty can often be marked by a worsening of the illness, so that young adults who had few problems as children can have repeated pain episodes.

Adult sickle-cell disease

Although most adults with sickle-cell disease have haemoglobin levels around 7 to 8 grams per decilitre, their worst problem – far greater than the fatigue of anaemia – is pain. It occurs in the torso and the limbs, and comes on suddenly, mostly without any obvious trigger. Cold can precipitate the pain: the literature describes arriving at a ski resort or swimming in cold water as pain-producers. Adults also suffer from acute chest problems, in which there is sudden onset of fever, breathlessness and cough: the cause is unknown, but it is not an infection. It is treated like asthma with bronchodilator drugs but, tragically, if no steps are taken to reverse the reaction the oxygen levels in the blood may fall, and death follows.

This severe and sudden chest reaction (it is called acute chest syndrome, or ACS) can be reversed by an exchange transfusion, in which all the patient's blood is passed through a pheresis machine. This acts like a filter to remove the abnormal haemoglobin thought to be the cause of the illness. If one is not available, then a straight blood transfusion can greatly improve the condition, especially if someone has started with a very low haemoglobin.

The most painful complication of adult sickle-cell disease is acute bone marrow necrosis. The pain is so severe in the ribs, the femur (thighbone) and tibia (shinbone) that many sufferers need epidural anaesthesia to control it. Patients who experience it say that it is far worse than their usual repeated pain episodes, and of a different quality. As with ACS, pheresis or exchange transfusion may be the only way to reverse the process. After bone marrow necrosis, the marrow's ability to produce red cells, already limited, is further reduced, so that the anaemia that accompanies every case of sickle-cell disease is worsened.

All the above complications are classified as acute, in that they arise suddenly, out of the blue. However, adults with sickle-cell disease must face many long-term problems. They include deterioration in their bones, so that long periods of standing become very painful; high blood pressure in the lungs due to repeated episodes of ACS (see above); and retinopathy (in which there is disease of the light-receptive screen at the back of the eye) that may lead to blindness. Every person with sickle-cell disease must have regular eye examinations to detect retinopathy as early in its development as possible, as it can be arrested in the early stages by laser treatment.

Treating sickle-cell disease

Apart from blood transfusion and pheresis in patients who are in desperate need of treatment for the acute episodes mentioned above, what can we do for sickle-cell anaemia? Many sickle-cell victims have the Multicenter Study of Hydroxyurea in Sickle Cell Anemia to thank for their improvement (Charache et al. 1995). Published in 1995, the study came to four main conclusions about hydroxyurea:

- It halves the numbers of pain crises.
- It halves hospital inpatient days for pain.
- It halves ACS (acute chest syndrome) instances.
- It significantly reduces the need for transfusions.

Best of all, it has been reported to lower the death rate in adult sickle-cell disease. It is now the standard treatment for people who are 18 years old or over (it is not yet approved for children), who are not pregnant and who have more than three pain crises a year, or have had a second attack of ACS, or need repeated transfusions.

Managing the pain in sickle-cell disease is a huge challenge. Because it is almost always present, patients need regular – usually daily – painkillers. However, taking daily prescription painkillers can damage the kidneys, so on top of all their health issues, people with sickle-cell anaemia have to have their kidney function checked regularly – remember the eGFR levels in the section in Chapter 6 on kidney disease? Adding kidney disease to a bone marrow that is already compromised by sickle disease poses considerable problems for the choice of treatment and for helping the patient avoid even more complications.

When the first-line painkillers prove not to be enough, the next stage in pain relief is to start on opiate-derived drugs. They do ease chronic pain, but at the price of dulling intellect and judgement and inducing tiredness. Worse, as sickle-cell disease is lifelong, opiates may need to be lifelong too, and this can lead to habituation and dependence on them. As a family doctor I can state definitively from experience that this presents us with one of the most difficult problems in patient management – how to keep someone lively and alert while treating his or her pain with long-term opiates.

Treating the anaemia

Blood transfusions are an essential in treating the anaemia in sickle-cell disease. Every person with sickle-cell disease is anaemic. Most have haemoglobin levels between 5 and 10 grams per decilitre, meaning that they have between one-third and two-thirds of the normal haemoglobin in the rest of the population. Simply giving iron does not help – a story that runs through the whole of this book – as the problem lies in the structure of the haemoglobin itself and not with iron deficiency. Transfusion of normal red cells can be lifesaving in crises, so it is an essential in particular cases. However, the physicians caring for people with the condition recognize that they must not push the haemoglobin level too high. If they raise the haemoglobin to levels of 11 or more grams per decilitre (well below the normal in the population) they risk blocking already damaged small arteries with the transfused cells. Most people with sickle disease are fairly comfortable with their usual haemoglobin level, even though well people would be extremely fatigued with it. Transfusions are therefore limited by most experts to people with haemoglobin levels around 5 grams per decilitre, as this is the level at which oxygen supply to the tissues starts to fall.

Repeated transfusions have been used in those with sickle-cell disease who have had strokes, in order to keep blood flow high through the brain, but they are less used for other complications. It is limited, however, by eventual transfusion reactions and by the build-up of iron, mentioned in previous chapters, that can lead to heart and liver failure. If iron overload has been unavoidable, it can be treated by desferrioxamine, given by slow intravenous drip over 12 hours, five days a week! Needless to say, this is an unpopular treatment.

Erythropoietin – again!

Recently erythropoietin, that useful treatment for kidney-related anaemia, has been tried in sickle disease with some success. This isn't surprising, as the kidneys deteriorate as the sickle cells block small arteries inside them and the eGFR falls. Giving one of the ESAs mentioned earlier can raise the haemoglobin by 2 or more grams per decilitre, and that can hugely improve people's sense of well-being.

Hydroxyurea can occasionally raise haemoglobin levels from around 7 to between 9 and 10 grams per decilitre, so it too is one of the options for improving the anaemia of many people with sickle-cell disease.

Stem cell transplantation

The real answer for them, however, is to try to establish a bone marrow in which the red cells are normal and the sickle-cell disease is cured. This is achieved by haematopoietic stem cell transplantation. The most suitable candidates for it are children with brothers or sisters whose blood is a match with theirs, but without the sickle-cell trait. The donor's stem cells, which will develop into cells that will produce normal red cells, are transplanted into the person's bone marrow once his or her own red cells have been removed.

It is hard to identify who is most suitable for transplant. Some people can manage to lead tolerable lives on the treatments described above; others have an exceptionally serious illness and will die early from it, but they need to be treated before they are too damaged by it to survive the process. It is a decision taken very seriously, and only by physicians extremely experienced in it.

Thalassaemia

Sickle cells are not the only way human beings found to combat malaria parasites. In 1925 Dr Thomas Cooley presented to the annual meeting of the American Pediatric Society the cases of five children with severe anaemia, enlarged spleens and odd bone abnormalities. They all had Italian or Greek backgrounds. Blood smears showed that they had abnormal red cells. In the next seven years doctors were finding other children with the same illness, many of them in countries around the shores of the eastern Mediterranean.

By 1932 the illness had been named thalassaemia, from the ancient Greek word for the sea.

Thalassaemia major

The affected children were extremely ill from their ninth month onwards, showing the same time of onset as sickle-cell disease, so that it became clear that the problem was with the type of their adult haemoglobin. As with sickling, it was only when their cells containing the normal foetal haemoglobin eventually disappeared from their bloodstream that the problems linked to possessing the abnormal haemoglobin arose.

The original children were seriously ill from the end of their first year onwards. They became paler and more irritable, grew more slowly than other children and became jaundiced. Their livers and spleens enlarged enormously as they tried to make more red cells to compensate for the anaemia. Even their facial bones tried to make blood, so that they expanded to produce very obviously different features.

Their red blood cells were pale, confirming that their haemoglobin levels were very low, at between 4 and 6 grams per decilitre. Many of the cells only had haemoglobin around their periphery, leading to their being called 'target' cells, after the appearance of an archery target. The reticulocyte count was raised to around 8 per cent, showing that the bone marrow was making an effort to compensate for the lack of haemoglobin, but the response was much lower than expected from such a severe anaemia.

The only treatment that could be offered was regular blood transfusion: without it, the children died before their fifth birthday. With transfusions, the children survived into their late teens; very few lived into their 20s. Their deaths were in part due to their anaemia, and in part due to the extra iron they had received from the transfused blood. A single unit of transfused blood contains 250 mg of iron, and the body cannot get rid of it, so over the years massive extra iron stores form in the child's liver, pancreas and especially the heart, where the scar tissue it produces eventually causes it to fail.

By the 1970s the children were being given hypertransfusions – very frequent transfusions aiming to keep the haemoglobin above 10 grams per decilitre. These had a dramatic effect, helping the children to be much more active physically and mentally and preventing the deformities of the face and bones, and the enlargements of the liver and spleen, that they would have otherwise had.

All children with this major form of thalassaemia are now managed with hypertransfusions from an early age. They enjoy a much more normal childhood but, sadly, the treatment has not prolonged their lives. The iron overload with its complications in the heart and the liver is still a life-limiting condition.

Lesser forms of thalassaemia – thalassaemia intermedia

Not all children with thalassaemia are as severely affected as those described above, who are classified as having thalassaemia major. Some children manage to maintain a haemoglobin of between 9 and 10 grams per decilitre. They feel better and are more active than children with the more severe disease, and they do not need repeated blood transfusions. A few patients can be converted from the major status to intermedia by removal of their spleen.

Why some children have the more severe and others the less severe form of the disease is not clear. To have either of them means that they have inherited two genes, one from each parent, and two children with ostensibly the same gene defects can be quite different in how much they are affected. As more than 150 separate mutations have already been described in the gene making just one of the components of haemoglobin in only one form of thalassaemia, it is clear that we have much more to learn about the subtle changes that each of them can initiate in the bone marrow.

Thalassaemia 'carriers'

Shortly after Dr Cooley's discovery, other investigators looked at relatives of those with the disease for clues to its cause. They found that close relatives did indeed have mild anaemias in which the red cells were much smaller than normal. However, this was all: otherwise they were living normal lives. It was clear that they were carriers of a single abnormal gene which gave rise to very minor changes in their blood-forming system. Further study confirmed that if two people with this form of anaemia had children together, the children were at very high risk (one in four) of developing the severe disease. The chances of this happening in populations with few people of Mediterranean background are rare, but not vanishingly so, as Greek and Italian communities tend to congregate together. Obviously they are much higher in Greece and Italy, so that it is common in these countries (and in other countries with communities in which there are many migrants from the eastern Mediterranean) for couples intending to marry to have genetic checks beforehand. Sadly, it is not unknown for intended marriages to be called off because of unfortunate test results.

This situation is even more difficult in people of Southeast Asian ancestry who have a slightly different form of thalassaemia from that common in the Mediterranean. Carriers of the single-gene defect of alpha-thalassaemia (the Mediterranean type is beta-thalassaemia) are completely normal: they don't show the small red cell type of mild anaemia. Many of them therefore do not suspect that they are carriers. With two gene mutations, they do show the mild anaemia and are classified as having 'alpha-thalassaemia trait'. Intermarriage of people who possess either type of gene mutation leads to a very high risk of severe thalassaemia in their children.

Treating thalassaemia

For thalassaemia major, the only current treatment is regular blood transfusions. Keeping the haemoglobin level at 10 grams per decilitre or more prevents the development of facial disfiguration and enlarged spleen and liver that makes life so intolerable for children with the condition.

In thalassaemia intermedia, the management is usually to 'watch and wait'. Most people with it manage reasonably well: their doctor's main worry is that they may worsen into a 'major' state. They therefore have to be monitored regularly to ensure that if their haemoglobin drops below 10 grams per decilitre they should start on regular transfusions. The balance must be weighed between the advantages of the higher haemoglobin and lesser disfigurement, and the disadvantage of inevitable long-term iron overload. Reducing iron load isn't a treatment to be taken lightly: it involves undergoing intravenous treatment for five days each week. Most people find it unpleasant, and some find it so intolerable that they refuse it, leaving themselves with a high risk of heart and liver problems.

People with thalassaemia trait need advice on the risks of their children inheriting a double genetic problem, with all that this implies for the major form of the illness.

9

Some less common anaemias

Haemolytic anaemia – Sylvia's case

Sylvia developed ulcerative colitis when she was 22. It was initially a stormy time for her, with several admissions as an emergency to hospital because of extreme abdominal pain and bouts of bloody diarrhoea. However, the disease settled on the usual treatment of steroid enemas and other anticolitis drugs, and for the next eight years she remained reasonably well, with only the occasional relapse that soon settled on emergency treatment.

It came as a surprise to us, as her doctors, when one day she attended the surgery complaining of weakness and tiredness, breathlessness, palpitations and dizziness, all of which had started only two weeks beforehand, when she was on holiday, and had worsened gradually since then. She had waited until she arrived back home before seeing a doctor, 'preferring the devils she knew to the ones she didn't'. We weren't sure that was a compliment.

It was immediately obvious that this was different from her previous bouts of colitis, because she had none of the abdominal pains or the diarrhoea that were the mainstays of all her earlier episodes of illness. Something she hadn't noticed, but that was very obvious to us, was that she had jaundice. The whites of her eyes were distinctly yellow and her skin was sallow. Her lips and nail beds were paler than both her doctors (I and a colleague) remembered from her previous visits to us. Listening to her chest, we both heard crackles at the bases of her lungs, suggesting fluid collecting there. This was of real concern, as it suggested heart failure.

Her 'spot' blood test showed a haemoglobin of only 6 grams per decilitre. As her previous haemoglobins were all around 12 grams per decilitre, she had obviously lost half her red blood cells in a very short time. How had this happened, when there had been no sign of bleeding? There was no blood in her stools or urine. This was obviously a case for our hospital physicians to sort out, urgently.

The microscopic appearance of her red cells made the diagnosis. There were two types of red cells in her blood: very small cells interspersed with a lower number of cells that were much larger than normal, inside which were lots of small dark bodies. The haematologist was in no doubt what the picture meant. The small cells were red cells stripped of their outer layer; the large cells were the reticulocytes mentioned in Chapter 1.

What was happening to Sylvia's blood? Her immune system was attacking her own red cells in the mistaken judgement that they were made of 'foreign' material. The red cells were haemolysing – breaking up and leaving free haemoglobin in the circulation, which was then 'mopped up' by the liver. In the process of coping with the extra haemoglobin, her liver was producing bilirubin, the yellow colour that gave her the jaundice and the sallow skin. The reticulocytes were her bone marrow's unsuccessful attempt to rectify the resulting anaemia, but as she had a haemoglobin of only 6 it was clear that the response was very much less than adequate.

Sylvia had immune haemolytic anaemia. It is a recognized complication of ulcerative colitis. We don't know exactly what it is about this illness that can turn the body against itself in this way, but ulcerative colitis isn't alone in doing so. It can occur in rheumatoid arthritis and in another inflammatory disease, systemic lupus erythematosus (SLE). It can complicate hepatitis C and HIV infections, and people with leukaemia, lymphoma and myeloma have a higher than normal risk of developing it. It can happen out of the blue in people with no previous illness. Very occasionally, it can be a side effect of a prescribed drug. The most common drug offender used to be the blood pressure-lowering agent methyldopa, but it is so seldom used nowadays that it is years since such cases were reported. The top spot for drugs that cause haemolytic anaemia is now occupied by a group of antibiotics called cephalosporins.

Not all cases of haemolytic anaemia are as dramatic as Sylvia's. There is a much milder form that may be found only by accident. People with it can keep their haemoglobin level between 10 and 11 grams per decilitre, and may not know they are anaemic until a spot check reveals it. The clue to their type of anaemia is their tiny round red cells, classified as microspherocytes: they are very deeply stained red because the haemoglobin is so concentrated within them.

Both types of haemolytic anaemia differ, too, from other forms of anaemia in that the jaundice is confirmed by high blood levels of the haemoglobin breakdown product bilirubin.

Treating haemolytic anaemia

Sometimes curing haemolytic anaemia is as simple as removing its cause – such as a cephalosporin. Usually, however, its treatment is much more difficult. The initial treatment of a severe case like Sylvia's involves using high doses of immune modulating drugs. Steroids are often the first choice, but newer approaches involve monoclonal antibody treatment, such as rituximab, and the cytotoxic agents cyclosporin A, cyclophosphamide and azathioprine. Another option is removal of the spleen.

Sylvia was given an intravenous drip containing immunoglobulin. Immunoglobulin attaches itself to the surface of the white cells that are destroying the red cells, stopping them from doing so. It is an immediate strategy that gives the physicians time to work out exactly which more long-term treatment will suit the patient. In extreme cases, they would have considered an exchange transfusion or pheresis, described in Chapter 8.

With this wide variety of treatments it may be plain to you that it takes real expertise to determine which is the appropriate one for each individual. The choice will surely be a matter for discussion by your hospital doctor team: it isn't in the remit of your general practitioner. However, there is one chink of encouragement for people with haemolytic anaemia: Sylvia recovered completely, and this is the usual experience, even when the illness has started so acutely and so severely.

Cold agglutinin anaemia – Margaret's case

Occasionally we can cure anaemia by making sure you wear a pair of warm gloves. Margaret reached her sixtieth birthday in perfect health. She had never had an operation, and prided herself in never having had to bother her doctor. From that birthday, in December, the pride became a fall. She started to have pains in her fingers, her ears, her nose and cheeks, and when the pain was at its height her skin in the same areas changed to a less than flattering dusky blue. The first attack had occurred on a very cold day, while she was walking her dog, but it persisted for several hours after getting warm at home. A friend told her she probably had Raynaud's disease and that nothing much could be done for it, so she delayed going to her doctor until the fourth attack, which happened at her daughter's house on Christmas Day. Their after-Christmas-lunch walk over a country track brought on an attack of extreme pain in her ears and nose (she was wearing warm gloves) that caused her to cry out. Her daughter, a nurse, took one look at the blue face and told her (she was that kind of daughter) that she must see the doctor at the first post-Christmas surgery.

Hearing the story on Boxing Day (I had drawn the short straw for duty that Christmas season) I was fairly sure that Margaret had cold agglutinin anaemia. I sent away a blood sample for testing, but the story she had told was typical enough for me to reassure her. The pains limited to the coldest parts of the body on the coldest days and the dusky blue colour (cyanosis) were clear evidence. Her age, too, was significant: 60 is the commonest age for it to start.

The blood picture confirmed the diagnosis. Her haemoglobin was only 10 grams per decilitre. The haematologist reported that some of her white cells had remnants of red cells inside them. The clincher for him was that when the red cells from the blood sample were exposed to the surface of a cold microscope slide, they clumped together – 'agglutinated' in medical parlance. Normal red cells don't do that.

People with cold agglutinin anaemia have in their blood high levels of a substance called IgM, or immunoglobulin M, which coats the red cells. The coating causes them to agglutinate when they are exposed to cold temperatures. The clumps of stuck-together red cells block very small arteries in the skin, depriving the areas beyond the blockages of oxygen. That causes the pain and the blue colour.

When this was explained to Margaret and she was advised to keep her skin warm in very cold weather (gloves, furry boots, ear muffs and woolly hoodie hats that protected her nose), she had no more attacks. Without her having to take iron, her haemoglobin gradually rose to 12.5 grams per decilitre. However, that wasn't the end of her story. Scotland isn't the warmest of places in the winter, and she had another daughter in Brisbane, Australia. She now spends half of her year in Oz and half in Scotland. I don't need to define which half for which country.

Fanconi's anaemia – a story of tragedy and triumph

I can't finish this book without paying tribute to three very special and courageous small boys and their devoted father. In the 1960s I was a house officer in Birmingham's Children's Hospital. Among my little patients were the three Collins brothers, Jimmy, Mark and David, aged 9, 11 and 14 respectively. They were super kids, normally full of fun, but often in pain and unhappy, especially when the day of their weekly blood transfusion came around.

All three boys had Fanconi's anaemia. In this terrible inherited disease the bone marrow slowly fails, so that it no longer makes enough white cells to fight off infection or red cells to maintain the body's oxygen needs. Affected children seem normal up to around age 7, but then the anaemia starts. They become ill from this time onwards, and die within three or four years. In the 1960s nothing could be done for them, except to give repeated blood transfusions that might give them a reasonable quality of life. For the Collins boys, transfusions were little help. Mark died in the August of my houseman year, Jimmy in the October, and David, who was old enough to know he was dying, struggled on to Christmas Day. I still remember them clearly more than 40 years later. I remember, too, their devoted dad, who had cared for them so lovingly (their mother had died before I met them) and who took his own life two weeks after David died.

This is a tragedy of which very few people have heard, but in 2012 it has a triumphant ending. In the last ten years our knowledge of, and ability to use, stem cells has improved so much that they can be used in medicine. Collected from bone marrow samples of unaffected siblings of children with Fanconi's anaemia, or even from their cord blood at birth, they transform into healthy blood-forming cells. Transplanted into the bone marrow of affected children, they form a healthy new blood-forming system producing all the white and red cells they need. Fanconi's anaemia was one of the first diseases in which the technique was spectacularly successful. The first treated Fanconi children are now healthy adults living completely normal lives. Many families have been spared the terrible experience of the Collins family.

There is so much hope for the future in today's medical research, not only for Fanconi anaemia but also for the many other lethal childhood anaemias that I have no room here to describe. I look forward with real optimism to a happier and healthier future for children and adults with every type of anaemia.

10

Some golden bullets

By now, having reached this far in the book, you will have gathered that anaemia is no simple matter to diagnose or to treat. You can't assume that if you feel tired or look pale you are anaemic. If you do find that you are anaemic, it is never enough to settle for iron supplements and 'wait and see' whether or not they work. So I am ending the book with a few 'golden bullets' on anaemia that will help you understand it and its management.

- Never assume, because you feel tired all the time, that you are bound to be anaemic.
- Don't be surprised if you are found to be anaemic even though you feel perfectly well.
- If you are found to be anaemic, accept that you must find out the cause before you simply take iron supplements.
- Most cases of anaemia are due to long-term bleeding from the bowel or from heavy menstrual periods, so be prepared, even if you haven't noticed bleeding, for your doctor to do tests before settling on the final treatment.
- If bleeding is found to be the cause of your anaemia, the source of the blood loss must be found and corrected. Your haemoglobin will then recover slowly over several months. You may be offered iron and vitamin supplements during the recovery months, but they are a temporary measure and never a substitute for cure of the cause. If you are normally healthy, eating a wide variety of foods, taking extra vitamins and minerals as supplements will not make you any

healthier and may be damaging to your long-term health. Mainstream medicine does not recommend vitamin supplements and minerals as a plan to prevent anaemia or other illnesses: it is always better for you to take in your daily requirements of them in what you eat.

- Iron treatment has a reputation for being simple and safe, but it is rare for it to be the whole answer to anaemia and it does not need to be continued beyond the time when your haemoglobin level is back to normal.

- If you have iron tablets or capsules in the house, never leave them within reach of young children. Even if there are no children in your home, remember that from time to time a visiting toddler might get hold of them. That could have tragic consequences: every doctor who has done a house job in a children's hospital will remember them.

- Even when you are anaemic, your body can't absorb more than a few milligrams of iron given as the usual tablets a day. You will absorb much more iron than from the tablets if you eat it in the form of red meat, because it is combined in haem, which your body uses a different pathway to digest.

- Repeated injections of iron, or repeated blood transfusions, have their drawbacks, in that the extra iron builds up to levels that may damage the liver and heart. So don't expect a 'quick fix' with them. If they are appropriate for you, your doctor will discuss your risks.

- For some anaemias, such as those linked to chronic kidney disease (affecting up to 10 per cent of people over 55), the appropriate treatment is erythropoietin (EPO), and not iron alone. But if you are given EPO you must eat healthily, with a wide variety of food containing all the nutrients needed for healthy red blood cells. You will need extra iron, but good food too.

- Anaemia can be one of the complications of other chronic

diseases, such as rheumatoid arthritis, coeliac disease, ulcer-ative colitis and cancer. Its causes in these illnesses are more complex than inability to digest iron or loss of blood: your doctor is now equipped to identify them and to correct them. Just because you have a long-term illness as well as your anaemia doesn't mean that the anaemia shouldn't be corrected. When it is, you will surely feel much better, even though your other illness continues on its course.

- In the Global North, vanishingly few people become anaemic because they do not eat sensibly. Foods contain-ing the essential nutrients needed for building up healthy red cells in their blood are widely available, and anyone eating a varied diet eats enough to keep a healthy marrow output of red cells. A very few extremely 'faddy eaters' who restrict themselves to a very narrow range of foods may become anaemic purely from missing out on essen-tial foodstuffs. They have to balance their decision on food restriction with their health needs. Taking iron and vitamin supplements and continuing on their poor diet is not the optimum answer for them. They need to eat foods contain-ing the proteins and fats for good bone marrow and other organ health, and their best choice is to consider changing their eating habits.

References

Bergmann, R. L. and colleagues (2002) 'Routine iron supplementation in pregnancy: why is the UK different?', *European Journal of Obstetrics and Gynaecology and Reproductive Biology*, 102: 155–60.

Bohlius, J., Wilson, J. et al. (2006) 'Recombinant human erythropoietin and cancer patients: updated meta-analysis of 57 studies including 9353 patients', *Journal of the National Cancer Institute*, 98: 708–14.

Bridges, Kenneth and Pearson, Howard A. (2008) *Anemias and Other Red Cell Disorders*, New York: McGraw Hill.

Charache, S., Terrin, M. L., Moore, R. D. et al. (1995) 'Effect of hydroxyurea on the frequency of painful crises in sickle-cell anemia', *New England Journal of Medicine*, 332: 1317–22.

Czeizel, A. E. and Dudas, I. (1992) 'Prevention of first occurrence of neural tube defects by periconceptional vitamin supplementation', *New England Journal of Medicine*, 327: 1832–5.

Delaby, C., Goncalves, A. S. et al. (2005) 'Presence of the iron exporter ferritin at the plasma membrane of macrophages is enhanced by iron loading and down-regulated by hepcidin', *Blood*, 106; 3979–84.

Eskes, T. (1997) 'Folates and the foetus', *European Journal of Obstetrics and Gynecology and Reproductive Biology*, 71: 105–11.

Frazer, D. M., Wilkins, S. J., Becker, E. M., Vulpe, C. D., McKie, A. T., Trinder, D. and Anderson, G. J. (2002) 'Hepcidin expression inversely correlates with the expression of duodenal iron transporters and iron absorption in rats', *Gastroenterology*, 123: 835–44.

Herrick, J. (1910) 'Peculiar elongated and sickle-shaped red blood corpuscles in a case of severe anemia', *Archives of Internal Medicine*, 6: 517–21.

Lozoff, B., Jimenez, E. and Wolf, A. W. (1991) 'Long-term developmental outcome of infants with iron deficiency', *New England Journal of Medicine*, 325: 687–94.

MRC Vitamin Study Research Group (1991) 'Prevention of neural tube defects: results of the Medical Research Council Vitamin Study (1991)', *The Lancet*, 338: 131–7.

Nilsson-Ehle, H., Swolin, B. and Westin, J. (1995) 'Bone marrow progenitor cell growth and karyotype changes in healthy 88-year-old subjects', *European Journal of Haematology*, 55: 14–18.

Olivares, M., Hertrampfl, E., Capurro, M. T. and Wegner, D. (2000) 'Prevalence of anemia in elderly subjects living at home: role of micronutrient deficiency and inflammation', *European Journal of Clinical Nutrition*, 54: 834–9.

Stone, P., Richardson, A. et al. (2000) 'Cancer-related fatigue: inevitable, unimportant and untreatable? Results of a multicentre patient survey', *Annals of Oncology*, 11: 971–5.

Taylor, D. J., Mallen, C. et al. (1982) 'Effect of iron supplementation of serum ferritin levels during and after pregnancy', *British Journal of Obstetric Gynaecology*, 89: 1011–17.

Timiras, M. and Brownstein, H. (1987) 'Prevalence of anemia and correlation of hemoglobin with age in a geriatric screening clinic population', *Journal of the American Geriatric Society*, 35: 639–43.

Index

acute chest syndrome (ACS) 83
alcoholism 4, 54
American Pediatric Society 87
anaemia, study in Germany 47–8
anaemia, types of *see individual anaemias*
angular stomatitis 18
anticonvulsants 55
anti-ulcer drugs 30–1
arthritis
 anaemia in 74–7
 rheumatoid 93, 100
atrophic glossitis (burning tongue) 18

Bridges, Dr Kenneth 25–7, 44, 80
British National Formulary 25–6

cancer
 bowel xv, 56
 Dundee University test 9
 oesophageal 39
cancer-related anaemia 77–9
cephalosporins 94
Charles II, King x
chronic inflammation, anaemia in (ACI) 74–7
coeliac disease 33–9, 100
 discovery of cause 37
coffee, and iron 32
 in pregnancy 32
cold agglutinin anaemia 95–7
Cooley, Dr Thomas 87, 90
C-reactive protein (CRP) 68–9
cytokines, inflammatory 75
cytotoxic agents 94

desferrioxamine 40–1

eGFR 69, 85
epilepsy 55
erythrocytes 1
erythropoiesis-stimulating agents (ESAs) 72–3, 77, 79, 86
erythropoietin (EPO) 71–4, 77, 86–7, 100

Fanconi's anaemia 97–8
 stem cell treatment in 98
ferritin 48
ferrous
 fumarate 26–7, 49
 gluconate 26–7, 49
 sulphate 26–7, 49
fibroids 15
fingernails 12
 see also koilonychia
foetal haemoglobin 81
folate deficiency 50
folic acid 50–6

gallstones 19
George III, King xvi
gluten 36–9

haematocrit 1
haemoglobin 1
haemolytic anaemia 92–5
hair changes 17
Helicobacter pylori 62
hepcidin 74–6
Herrick, Dr James 80
hydroxyurea 87
hypertransfusions 89
hysterectomy 15

immunoglobulin 94–6
inflammatory bowel disease xvi

Ingram, Dr Vernon 81
iron deficiency, teenage 22
iron injections 49
iron-deficiency anaemia 23

kidney disease (CKD) 67–73
koilonychia 16, 34
    see also fingernails

leukaemia 94
leukocytes 1
lymphoma 94

meat, red 28
Medical Research Council 81
monoclonal antibody treatment 94
myeloma 94

older people, anaemia in 64–7

Paterson-Brown-Kelly syndrome 35
Pearson, Dr Howard A. 25–7, 44, 80
periods, heavy 12–13
pernicious anaemia xii, xv, 56–63
Plummer-Vinson syndrome 35,
    38–9
pregnancy 25, 43
prostate health test (PSA) 68

reticulocytes x, 10

Shaw, George Bernard 54, 66
sickle-cell anaemia 80–7

signs of serious illness 11, 18
spina bifida 51
spleen 82, 94
stem cell transplantation 87
steroids 94
stomach
    surgery 63
    ulcers xvi
Stone, Dr P. 78
systemic lupus erythematosus (SLE)
    93

tannin 32
tea 30–6
thalassaemia 87–91
tinnitus 60
transferrin 46–8
transfusions 86

ulcerative colitis 95, 100
ultrasound tests 14
United Kingdom 25, 47, 67, 80
United States 25, 47, 80

vegetarians 101
vitamin A 61
vitamin B12 xv, 4, 58–63
vitamin C 26–8
vitiligo 61

well-man clinic xvi, 9, 10, 11, 18,
    68
well-woman clinic xvi, 6, 8

Printed in Great Britain
by Amazon.co.uk, Ltd.,
Marston Gate.